mind over matter

Susan Cantwell

mind over matter

Personal Choices for a Lifetime of Fitness

Foreword by Silken Laumann

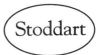

Copyright © 1999 by Susan Cantwell

All rights reserved. No part of this publication may be reproduced or transmitted in any form or by any means, electronic or mechanical, including photocopying, recording, or any information storage and retrieval system, without permission in writing from the publisher.

Published in 1999 by Stoddart Publishing Co. Limited
34 Lesmill Road, Toronto, Canada M3B 2T6
180 Varick Street, 9th Floor, New York, New York 10014

Distributed in Canada by:
General Distribution Services Ltd.
325 Humber College Blvd., Toronto, Ontario M9W 7C3
Tel. (416) 213-1919   Fax (416) 213-1917
Email customer.service@ccmailgw.genpub.com

Distributed in the United States by:
General Distribution Services Inc.
85 River Rock Drive, Suite 202, Buffalo, New York 14207
Toll-free Tel. 1-800-805-1083   Toll-free Fax 1-800-481-6207
Email gdsinc@genpub.com

03   02   01   00   99   1   2   3   4   5

Canadian Cataloguing in Publication Data

Cantwell, Susan
Mind over matter: personal choices for a lifetime of fitness

ISBN 0-7737-3216-0

1. Exercise. 2. Physical fitness. 3. Health. I. Title.

RA781.C36 1999   613.7   C99-931459-9

Jacket design: Bill Douglas @ The Bang
Design and typesetting: Kinetics Design & Illustration

THE CANADA COUNCIL | LE CONSEIL DES ARTS
FOR THE ARTS | DU CANADA
SINCE 1957 | DEPUIS 1957

We acknowledge for their financial support of our publishing program the Canada Council, the Ontario Arts Council, and the Government of Canada through the Book Publishing Industry Development Program (BPIDP).

Printed and bound in Canada

To my husband, Derrick,

for his never-ending encouragement and support

and to our three children, Nicholas, Alexandria, and Max

— who give new meaning to the phrase "active living."

And to my mother:

thanks for always being there

even before I know I need you.

Contents

Acknowledgements

$\mathcal{I}$ would like to thank Stephen Quick and all the great people at Stoddart Publishing, who believed in this book from the beginning.

My thanks also go out to Kathy Bockus, Rhona Sawlor, and Rosemary Ogilvie, Connie Petrie, Peter Kaufman, Randy Withrow, and Barbara Harris.

And, finally, thanks to Silken Laumann, Dr. Susan Bartlett, Dr. James Prochaska, Sophie Giountsis-Turner, Maureen Hagan, Sharon Porter, Amanda Hanbidge, Beth Rothenberg, Marjorie O'Conner, Donna Read, and Gary McCoy for their time, support, and advice.

$\mathcal{F}$oreword

$\mathcal{T}$his is not just another diet book. This is not a book about following a sixty-day program and emerging twenty pounds thinner. This is a book about positive lifestyles and how to tap into the underlying goals and motivations that make change possible.

In *Mind Over Matter* Susan Cantwell encourages each of us to uncover our own passionate reasons for wanting to change our lifestyles. Most people say they want to exercise to lose weight or to look better, but when they start to examine their motivations more closely they find a whole slew of reasons to start exercising and eating well. They may hope to reduce their chances of following in the footsteps of a parent who died of a heart attack at a young age, to find more energy, or to regain a sense of control.

Certainly, as an athlete, the most common questions I am asked are about motivation and goal setting. People want to know how they can motivate themselves to get up every morning to exercise; they want to know the secret discipline to choosing carrot sticks over potato chips. I am struck by how often people tell me they don't have enough self-discipline to change their lifestyle. I have more faith in people than that. Most people *do* have self discipline, they *can* motivate themselves; but as Susan points out, they often lack commitment and a sound understanding of what they need to do to make change happen.

In this book Susan helps you develop a plan for success. She asks you to examine whether you are ready to change, to determine why you want to change, to foresee your obstacles, and to develop strategies that work for you. Each chapter includes a real-life case study, so real that you will see yourself in a few of them.

Many fitness programs and diets are unrealistic in the long term. They often don't take into account the time pressures of our busy lives. Susan's suggestions are not about what to eat, or how long to exercise, they are about how to structure our lives to make eating well and exercising possible. Her realistic analysis is refreshing, and by the end of the book we have the definite feeling that fitness is something we can achieve.

My good friend Carmen wants to get fit and lose weight. Since giving birth a year ago she has carried twenty extra pounds. She stays at home with her daughter three days a week; she runs a small business on two others. Between working, running her household, and looking after her daughter she can't find the time to exercise. She wants to lose weight but each time she starts to eat sensibly she actually gains weight. Last week she asked me to recommend a good diet and exercise book. I will send her a copy of *Mind Over Matter* as soon as it is in print. This book will show her that her problem is not a lack of discipline or motivation, it is a lack of planning. She hasn't set herself clear reasons for changing her lifestyle and she hasn't anticipated the inevitable obstacles. When we say we want to eat well, most of us don't factor in the time needed to prepare healthy meals and the planning that needs to go into making a shopping list. Although we want to exercise more, most of us haven't prepared a plan of what to do if our children are sick on the evening we planned to exercise, or if it is raining when we planned to go cycling. This lack of planning inevitably leads to feelings of failure.

In my life as an athlete, staying fit and healthy was my full-time job. I didn't have to give a second thought to maintaining my ideal weight or exercising regularly. But since retiring from rowing I have started a family and am running a full-time business, both of which put such heavy demands on my time that eating well and exercising regularly have become a real challenge. After a day at work, I am reluctant to leave my son while I go rowing.

I have found that I, like most working parents, need to cultivate a spirit of compromise. My family goes for long walks together, and we have purchased a bicycle trailer so we can spend time together while getting fresh air and exercise. I would often rather be out rowing, but that isn't always possible.

In short, I am facing the same challenge most of us face: making the time to exercise and eat well. I found reading *Mind Over Matter* a good reminder of how to make it all work. I have renewed confidence that our busy family will live an active and healthy lifestyle. One of the greatest gifts we can give our children is time spent together; when this time is active time it is all the more rewarding. I hope to be playing soccer with my son well into my sixties, and ultimately I hope that through our experiences as an active family he will gain an appreciation for physical activity and healthy eating. Eating well and staying active are key to health and happiness.

Silken Laumann

*P*reface

I have been a lifestyle consultant and personal trainer for over ten years. During these ten years, I began to notice common problems that people share when trying to start and stick to their lifestyle changes. I began documenting these problems. For all of the hundreds of clients I have worked with over the years, the missing link was preparation. How you prepare yourself mentally before starting to exercise and eat properly plays a large role in determining whether you will be successful. *Mind Over Matter* brings together all the information you will need to successfully change your exercise or eating habits, and gives you a clear path to follow.

In this book, you will notice that there are many references to weight loss. I focused on this particular problem because people tend to struggle with their weight year after year. The goal of *Mind Over Matter* is to help you to lead a healthier and happier life — permanently. You can take the information in this book and apply it to any health-related goal you may have.

I wish you the best of luck on your journey to better health.

Susan Cantwell
March 1999

1

Laying the Foundation for Success

$\mathcal{E}$veryone wants to be healthy, feel good, and look attractive. Everyone wants to live a long life, have plenty of energy, and enjoy what life has to offer. One of the main components of living life to the fullest is leading a healthy lifestyle, which includes exercising and eating properly. If we do not exercise regularly and eat a proper diet, we can never truly achieve mental and physical well-being. Feeling good about the way we look — with all the advantages or disadvantages our genes have passed on to us — has a direct effect on how we feel about ourselves. And how we feel about ourselves plays a part in our ability to successfully implement healthy changes in our lives.

Looking and feeling good means different things to different people. Looking good to a small person might mean gaining five or ten pounds; to a larger person it might mean losing them. Everyone has different goals and motivations. For some, feeling good might involve reducing stress and having more energy to do the things they enjoy after they have put in an eight-hour work day. For others, feeling positive about the way they look and having the confidence to take on new challenges might be the key. But all of us, large or small, strong or weak, tired or energetic, need to exercise and eat a proper diet to reach our full potential. Whatever our goals, the challenge remains the same: how to eat properly and exercise consistently to reach those goals.

Many people struggle with weight issues. Poor eating habits and a lack of exercise can increase our weight in just a short time. Remember the days when you could eat and drink anything you wanted and not put on an ounce?

At thirty-something, you probably started to notice that you were not burning off calories the way you used to. There is a good reason for this. After thirty or so, the average sedentary person's metabolism slows, due to the loss of muscle. In ten years of decreasing muscle mass, you could gain almost ten pounds without eating more or decreasing your activity level.

The North American weight-loss industry reported a whopping $33 billion in revenues in 1997. At any given time, 62 percent of adults in North America are trying to lose weight, most not for the first time. We all know that we need to exercise and eat properly. So why is it so hard to do?

Every time a new diet book or program comes out, we flock to it; we didn't stick with the last one, but the new one must be better. Let's face it, there's no shortage of methods — books, pills, drinks, and programs — designed to help us become more healthy. While some of these programs are more credible than others, the best method is one we can stick to over a lifetime.

Many people feel discouraged when they try to start exercising and eat properly, only to revert to their former bad habits. "Why can't I do it?" they wonder. "What is wrong with me? Is it a lack of willpower, or am I just lazy?" Certainly not! Most of us who fail to reach our goals and stay there permanently fail because the most crucial step on the road to implementing healthy change is the one we most often overlook. This key step, or phase, should be taken before we ever put on a pair of running shoes or buy the newest diet book. So what is this crucial phase? I call it the pre-planning or preparation phase, and it's the foundation on which success is built.

Imagine that you are building a house and you pay little attention to the quality of the foundation. Instead you decide to spend a lot of money on paint finishes and interior decorating. After a period of time your foundation begins to crack, shift, and crumble. What happens to the beautifully decorated floors, walls, and ceilings?

The same thing may happen to you if you try to bring exercise and healthy eating habits into your life without properly preparing yourself and the people around you for these changes. Your good intentions will crack, shift, and eventually crumble. Preparation is the essential first step on your path to good health.

How We Think Affects How We Feel

*I*f you have ever exercised in a fitness facility, you may have noticed that all the parking spaces right in front of the facility's doors are always taken. Members drive into the parking lot and circle the spaces in front looking for the perfect parking space. They'll even wait five or ten minutes for someone to pull out before they give up and park in a space across the lot. Disgruntled, they enter the facility complaining about the lack of parking spaces out front. Then they get on a treadmill to walk for thirty minutes!

People who can relate to this scenario have not made the mental connection between exercise programs and an active lifestyle. Their chances of reaching their personal fitness goals and maintaining healthy habits are slim.

To change your lifestyle permanently, you must view proper eating and regular exercise not as seasonal activities, but as a year-round way of life. A seasonal mentality is evident in the yearly cycle of the fitness club industry. September and January bring the largest influx of new members and revenue; the summer months and December bring the biggest drop-off in attendance.

To anyone who is trying to lose weight, the word "diet" is indeed a four-letter word. Diet has been made to mean something that it does not mean. A diet is a selection of foods. You can eat a diet full of vegetables and fruits or you can eat a diet of cheeseburgers and chocolate. But to many people, being "on a diet" is synonymous with feeling deprived, going hungry, and counting calories. The start of a diet can bring on feelings of apprehension, resignation, and martyrdom. These negative emotions often result in a pre-diet binge. Once D-Day (diet day one) has been set, the dieters start to increase the intake of foods they most fear being deprived of during their "diet." People who would normally choose not to order a dessert in a restaurant now order pie and ice cream, with the rationalization, "Oh well, I am going on a diet on Monday." (Most people will pick Monday to begin a change in their eating habits because it is the first day in a new week — but also so that they can have that last weekend hurrah!)

The exercise on the next page illustrates that how we think about our lifestyle changes is vital to how motivated we are to make them.

For each of the following questions, write down the first three words that come to mind.

A How do you feel about the word "diet"?

1 ....

2 ....

3 ....

B How do you feel the about the phrase "healthier eating habits"?

1 ....

2 ....

3 ....

A How do you feel about the word "exercise"?

1 ....

2 ....

3 ....

B How you do feel about the words "active living"?

1 ....

2 ....

3 ....

Are your answers to the "A questions" more negative than those for the "B questions"? When we begin exercising and trying to eat better with a negative mindset, we often must force ourselves to actually *do* what we know we should.

You can only feel good about — and stick to — your lifestyle changes if you approach them in the right frame of mind. Positive actions flow from a positive outlook. Successful change is a marriage of intellect and emotion, with action being the "child" that results from that marriage.

Negative Dynamic

The Intellect: I want to get in shape and lead a healthier lifestyle.
I know I need to do this, but it is a lot of work.

The Emotion: I am afraid of change, afraid of failure, and apprehensive in general.

The Action: I have done nothing, procrastinating for a time.

Positive Dynamic

The Intellect: I am going to get into shape and follow a healthier lifestyle.
I will do this. I am willing to put in the effort that making changes in my life will require.

The Emotion: I am relieved, optimistic, and excited.

The Action: I have started to exercise and eat a healthy diet.

Time and Consistency = Results and Motivation

Whatever the century or fashion, people have been trying to lose weight, get in shape, and feel better about themselves. Marie Antoinette's comment, "Let them eat cake" was said through a mouthful of crumbs. She had just fallen off the diet wagon and wanted her courtiers to join her. When Julius Caesar said, "Et tu, Brute?" he was sympathizing with his ally's unsuccessful attempt to stick to his exercise program.

Of course, these versions of the two famous historical anecdotes are not accurate. Marie Antoinette and Caesar were probably far too proud to tell anyone that they could not stick with their lifestyle changes.

Timing Is Everything

Research shows that the three main reasons people say they are unable to stick with an exercise program and eat properly are lack of time, poor motivation, and unsatisfactory results. When we begin a fitness program, our resolve is usually strong. Why doesn't it remain so?

Life gets in the way: appointments, work, children, parents, responsibilities, and obligations take up most of our time. Results lie in consistency. It takes time to plan healthy meals and it takes time to exercise. Many of us begin a fitness program and promise we will change our eating habits but do not allow time in our schedules to accommodate our resolutions.

How often does this scenario happen? You are late getting home from work, your family is hungry, and nothing is prepared. You can either fix a quick veggie platter with dip for the kids while you prepare a healthy meal or order takeout food. Most of us pick up the phone and order in. Convenience wins out because no time has been built into our daily schedules to allow for the necessary changes in lifestyle that healthy eating and exercise require.

When something becomes inconvenient, but we know we should still do it, we experience anxiety, guilt, and resentment. When faced with two choices, the path of least resistance becomes well travelled. When we do not allocate the time needed to build the proper foundation for our goals, we cannot put up walls to support the floors and staircases that take us to the next level.

The charts on pages 10–12 are designed to help you evaluate your weekly schedule and allocate time to exercise and eat properly. You can change them weekly as your schedule changes.

First, block off your work hours. If you work at home taking care of preschool children, block off all the hours that are non-nap times. Next, fill in any activities, in the day or evening, that you *must* be available for, such as driving a child to a hockey practice, attending a doctor's appointment, helping out in play group, and so on. Next, block off any social obligations such as committee work, volunteer duties, dinner parties, or family get-togethers. Remember to allow yourself an hour before you go to bed to unwind from your hectic day.

When you are finished filling in this form, you will be able to see where in your schedule you can comfortably find time to implement your lifestyle changes. The next step is to find three hours a week to exercise and two to five hours a week for meal planning and meal preparation, a total of five to eight hours a week. If you feel discouraged when you look at your schedule, remember that there are 168 hours in a week. Subtracting eight hours for sleep each night still leaves a total of 112 waking hours. Remember: even if you lead an especially busy life, when something important comes up, you always find time to take care of it. Now is the time to let your health and well-being assume the same importance.

Schedule your exercise time first. If you have not exercised in a while, or are a beginner, you should plan for one hour, two to three days a week. Don't expect to exercise for a full hour right off the top. The hour provides a cushion of time for travel and getting ready, and allows you to slowly increase the number of minutes you exercise as you become more fit.

The next thing you need to do is to plan when you are going to change your eating habits. ***You do not have to start exercising and eating properly during the same week***. Before trying to change your eating habits, you should keep a Food Journal for seven consecutive days to see the pattern of what you eat and when you eat. This Food Journal provides a record of everything you eat and drink, including snacks, during a seven-day period. The point is *not* to change your eating habits during this week, only to record them. After you complete your Food Journal, sit down and review what you ate, at what time of day, what you were doing, and what you were feeling. Many people are surprised by what they see.

A sample Food Journal for you to fill in appears on page 12.

Next, plan your menu. Decide what you and your family are going to eat for the next seven days. That includes breakfast, lunch, dinner, a snack in the morning, and a snack in the afternoon. If you feel that you cannot plan your menu seven days in advance, start by planning at least two days in advance. This will give you time to practise and perfect your planning. Once you find two days easy to plan, extend the number of days to five and then to seven.

Scheduling for Success

Time	Monday	Tuesday	Wednesday
6:00 AM			
6:30 AM			
7:00 AM			
7:30 AM			
8:00 AM			
8:30 AM			
9:00 AM			
9:30 AM			
10:00 AM			
10:30 AM			
11:00 AM			
11:30 AM			
12:00 PM			
12:30 PM			
1:00 PM			
1:30 PM			
2:00 PM			
2:30 PM			
3:00 PM			
3:30 PM			
4:00 PM			
4:30 PM			
5:00 PM			
5:30 PM			
6:00 PM			
6:30 PM			
7:00 PM			
7:30 PM			
8:00 PM			
8:30 PM			
9:00 PM			
9:30 PM			
10:00 PM			

Thursday	Friday	Saturday	Sunday

Food Journal

		Food	Time	Activity	Feelings
Mon	Breakfast				
	Snack				
	Lunch				
	Snack				
	Dinner				
	Snack				
Tues	Breakfast				
	Snack				
	Lunch				
	Snack				
	Dinner				
	Snack				
Wed	Breakfast				
	Snack				
	Lunch				
	Snack				
	Dinner				
	Snack				
Thurs	Breakfast				
	Snack				
	Lunch				
	Snack				
	Dinner				
	Snack				
Fri	Breakfast				
	Snack				
	Lunch				
	Snack				
	Dinner				
	Snack				
Sat	Breakfast				
	Snack				
	Lunch				
	Snack				
	Dinner				
	Snack				
Sun	Breakfast				
	Snack				
	Lunch				
	Snack				
	Dinner				
	Snack				

When you know what you are going to eat, it will be easier to stick to your diet changes. You can also shop for what you need to prepare these meals, so you are sure to have the necessary ingredients in the house. If there are always healthy choices available, there will be less temptation to slip off the wagon "just this once."

You have now allocated the *time* in your schedule to allow you to exercise and eat properly. If you do not put your plan in writing, another activity may all too easily take priority. We who lead busy lives with many demands placed on our time must balance future needs with present ones. Because our present needs have immediate consequences, we tend to minimize the long-term effects that our present behaviours will have on our health. Every time we choose not to exercise or eat properly, we are closing our eyes to the possible consequences, and gambling with our future.

The Weight-loss Merry-Go-Round

Another major factor in your ability to reach your goals is **consistency**. If you do not exercise and eat properly on a consistent basis, will you get the results you want? No. How will you feel if you get minimal results and do not reach your initial goals? Most people become demotivated and their level of consistency drops even further. Many then give up and revert to their previous habits. This cycle is all too familiar:

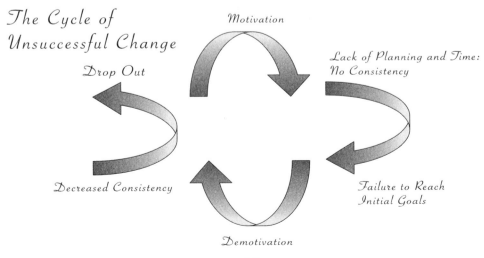

The Cycle of Unsuccessful Change

Motivation

Lack of Planning and Time: No Consistency

Drop Out

Decreased Consistency

Failure to Reach Initial Goals

Demotivation

As you can see, planning your time has a direct effect on whether you will be able to eat properly and exercise consistently. Consistency has a direct effect on whether you will reach your initial goals. When you fail to reach your initial goals, you become demotivated about continuing to eat properly and exercise. Your consistency flags and eventually you abandon your plans to change your lifestyle.

If you have tried before to stick with a fitness program and were not successful, identify at which point in the cycle you experienced the most difficulty. Then look at the previous arrow; your troubles might actually have begun there.

You must follow the Cycle of Success in order to reach your goals:

The Cycle of Success

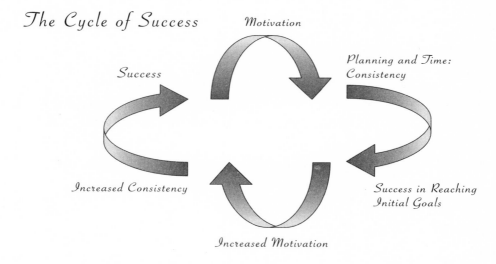

Motivation

Planning and Time: Consistency

Success

Increased Consistency

Success in Reaching Initial Goals

Increased Motivation

Once you understand the importance of and the relationships among time, consistency, results, and motivation, you are well on your way to avoiding the merry-go-round of repeated attempts to change your lifestyle. You will be able to sidestep the negative emotions that come with perceived failure, such as self-doubt and declining self-confidence.

An understanding of what is required helps you to commit yourself to the lifestyle changes you have chosen and to make these changes a reality. One way to commit yourself is to draw up a Participation Agreement, or self-contract. Take a few minutes to read over the self-contract below. You will want to photocopy it and personalize the contract to suit your needs and goals.

Participation Agreement

I, ..., will make exercise a priority in my life.

1. I will exercise a minimum of .... hours a week.
2. I will exercise on ...., ..., and .... at these times, ..., ..., and ....
3. I understand that I may have to modify or change my eating habits.
4. I will schedule time in my day to eat properly.
5. I understand that I may have to make lifestyle changes in keeping with my commitment to lead a healthy lifestyle.
6. I understand that I am responsible for reaching my goals and that what I do in all aspects of my life can affect my overall health.
7. I know that I am worth the effort it will require to lead a happy and healthy lifestyle.

Personal Commitments

1 ....

2 ....

3 ....

Date: .... Signature: ....

You have just made a promise to yourself *in writing*. Display it in a place where you will see it every day, perhaps in a picture frame beside your bed, taped to your fridge, or placed in your briefcase on top of your work.

Case Study *Good Intentions*

Donna has reached a phase of her life when she feels she should be quite content. At forty-eight, she no longer needs to work and her husband owns a thriving computer company. Her two children, Alex, fourteen, and Rose, sixteen, are excelling academically and socially. Donna has many friends and she and her husband lead active social lives. They go to fundraisers and school functions for their children, and often have a weekly invitation to go out for dinner with friends. But Donna doesn't "feel good." Each time she has to go out, she dreads looking in her closet for something to wear. Once she finally decides on an outfit and does her hair and make-up she usually perks up, but out among other people she feels self-conscious. Her clothing is getting tight and she knows she will soon need a larger size.

When did I put on all this weight? she wonders. Donna goes into the bathroom and weighs herself: 165 pounds. She is shocked; she has never weighed that much before.

She decides to change her eating habits and start exercising. Her first step is to buy an exercise bike. She puts it in the television room so she can exercise while watching her favourite shows. Her second step is to pick a date to start her diet: the following Monday. Donna decides to exercise during the day when the kids are at school. She feels optimistic and looks forward to gaining control of her weight.

The weekend before Donna plans to start her diet, she and her husband join another couple at one of their favourite restaurants. Donna orders steak and a baked potato with butter and sour cream. She starts with a Caesar salad that she knows has a lot of calories and fat compared with the green salad she usually orders. *Oh well*, she thinks, *this is the last chance I have to eat like this for a while.*

After dinner, Donna orders chocolate cheesecake.

"You don't usually order dessert," her husband remarks.

"Oh, every once in a while I just feel like something sweet." Donna smiles, and everyone decides to order dessert. For the rest of the weekend,

Donna abandons all restraint. If her kids are eating potato chips, she helps herself. She makes a rich Sunday dinner, complete with cream sauces and plenty of butter.

On Monday morning, Donna wakes up feeling motivated. After she feeds the kids and gets them off to school, she decides that instead of a bagel with cream cheese and a bowl of fruit, she'll have just the bowl of fruit. She then throws herself into vigorously cleaning the house. She glances at her exercise bike as she vacuums the television room. *I'll exercise this afternoon,* she decides. At 12:30 Donna rushes to a fund-raiser luncheon at a nearby hotel.

At the luncheon, Donna and other committee members talk about various ideas for raising money for their local chapter of the Heart Foundation. Donna stays away from the foods she knows are high in fat, but eats a large lunch. Only after she leaves does she realize how hungry she had been and how much she ate as a result.

Donna gets home at 3:00. She still has an hour to exercise before the kids arrive. Donna is heading for her room to get changed when she remembers that she has to take the clothes from the washer and put them in the dryer. She then stops in the kitchen to take some chicken out of the fridge to defrost for supper. It is 3:30 when she heads upstairs to change. As Donna comes down, the telephone starts to ring. It's her brother, who wants to know what she is going to get for their parents' thirty-eighth wedding anniversary the following weekend. Just as she puts the telephone down, her kids walk through the door.

"Alex, get a snack. You have hockey practice in half an hour. Rose, are you coming?" Donna yells as she starts back up the stairs to change again.

"No, I'm going to Sarah's house," Rose says, as she opens the fridge.

"All right, be home for six o'clock for supper," Donna replies.

Donna gets her son to the rink by 4:30. As she watches him practise, she decides to exercise right after supper.

Donna pulls into her driveway at the same time her husband does. It's now 6:00. She immediately starts preparing supper while her husband changes.

I will make chicken, broccoli with cheese sauce, and rice. I just won't have the cheese sauce, thinks Donna. While she's cutting up the cheese for the sauce, she pops a few pieces into her mouth. By the time she's finished, she's eaten several chunks.

Supper is ready by 6:45, a bit later than usual, but that's not unusual on the days Alex has hockey. It's 7:45 by the time Donna has eaten, cleaned up the kitchen, and sat down with her husband to have a cup of tea. Donna calls to her children, "Do you guys have any homework?"

"Yes," they both answer.

"Get started," she urges. After twenty minutes, Alex calls from the kitchen, "Mom, I need you!" Donna often helps Alex with math and rather enjoys it. In the meanwhile, Donna's husband has agreed to drive Rose to a friend's house to work on a school project.

At 8:30 Donna finishes helping her son with his homework and tells him to go upstairs to take a shower. She goes back into the kitchen to start making lunches for her children for the following day. The telephone rings for her husband. There's a problem about a presentation that her husband's company is giving the next day. Before he takes the call, he asks if she can pick up Rose at her friend's house at 9:30 since the phone call might take a while.

At 10:15 Donna comes back downstairs after saying good night to the kids and heads for the laundry room to take the clothes out of the dryer. She folds them in the television room while she and her husband watch the television.

"Did you use your bike today?" he asks.

"No. I didn't get a chance, but I'll start tomorrow," Donna vows.

Donna doesn't get on the bike until Wednesday and then only for fifteen minutes before she has to get ready for a doctor's appointment. She continues to cook her family's regular meals and but doesn't eat anything she thinks is high in fat, although she still picks at food while she is preparing it. On Thursday, Donna's legs are stiff and sore from exercising on Wednesday. She decides to skip a day because her legs hurt too much but determines to get back on the bike on Friday.

On Friday night, Donna is proud that she managed to bike for twenty minutes. She was extremely busy all day, following up on last-minute arrangements for her parents' anniversary party.

Saturday is crazy. The telephone rings constantly. Donna cleans the entire house with the help of her kids. At 5:00 the caterers arrive and her husband leaves to pick up the cake. Donna runs upstairs to shower and change.

The evening is a success. Everyone raves about the food and has a good time. Donna and her husband see the last of the guests out at 1:30 a.m. She believes she has stuck to her diet pretty well — after all, it *was* her parents' anniversary party. Besides, she watched what she was eating the entire week before the party.

Donna wakes up Sunday morning tired and with a slight headache. There's still some cleaning up to do from the night before. Her husband's busy making a brunch, of sorts, from the leftover food. Donna eats a bit as she drinks her coffee. *Exercise today?* she thinks. *No way. I am too tired.*

On Monday morning Donna gets on the scale and looks down in anticipation. She exercised twice the previous week and watched what she ate for the most part. But she cannot believe what she sees. One hundred and sixty-seven pounds — two pounds *more* than she weighed the previous week! She jumps off the scale and goes downstairs to watch television. As she enters the room she glances at the exercise bike. *I have a very busy week coming up. If I can find the time, I'll exercise*, she thinks, before turning on the TV.

The next week is so hectic she manages to get on the bike for only fifteen minutes on one day. The following Monday she weighs herself: still 167 pounds. The week after, she can't find the time to exercise at all.

Donna's exercise bike is eventually brought up to her bedroom. Her husband complains that she has wasted three hundred dollars. Donna jokes that it's an expensive clothes hanger.

Donna feels worse about herself than she did before she started trying to diet and exercise. Her self-esteem has dwindled and she wonders why she doesn't have the willpower to stick to what she started.

But Donna does not lack willpower. What she lacks is a specific plan to incorporate her lifestyle changes into her life. With better planning, she could have realized many health-related returns for investing in an exercise bike. She can still lose the weight she wants, if she plans a specific time to exercise and organizes her menus so that the whole family eats the same healthy foods. Donna also needs to examine why she puts her own needs last, as she rushes around to help her kids, her husband, and the other people who make demands on her time.

Ten Key Steps to Success

Life is full of change. Some changes we cannot anticipate, but others we can. When we actively participate and seek change in our lives, we take responsibility for and control of our lives. In trying to improve our health, we are making connections among our intellect, our emotions, and our actions. Some refer to this process as making the mind-body connection.

If you have tried to start exercising and eating properly before and have failed, do not despair that you will not reach your goals this time. This time you are taking the steps to build a strong foundation for success.

1 Remember that the pre-planning or preparation phase is the most crucial part of any lifestyle change.

2 Make the connection between your mind and your body. The fulfillment of your goals depends on this connection.

3 Examine your feelings about diet, exercise, and change. Are these feelings hindering you or helping you?

4 Plan for success by allocating time to exercise and eat properly, and make appointments with yourself in writing.

5 Remember the relationships among time, consistency, results, and motivation. Without the first, the others cannot be achieved.

6 Pick a date when you will begin exercising and write it down.

7   Choose a date that is seven days from this date to begin changing your eating habits. During these seven days, keep a Food Journal to record what you are eating, when you are eating it, what you are doing, and how you are feeling.

8   Make a written contract with yourself that outlines your personal expectations.

9   Plan in advance what you will eat for each meal, including snacks.

10   Commit to taking responsibility for and control of your health before you begin a program.

2

Are You Ready to Change?

*W*hen you decide that you want to make lifestyle changes, your initial motivation may come from an external source: a concerned spouse, a close friend, or a new policy at work, for example. But if you are not ready to change, your chances of succeeding are slim. When you feel pushed towards change rather than motivated by your own internal resolution, you most likely will not make your best effort. If you are not committed to lifestyle changes, you cannot succeed, and your failure will reinforce any doubts you might have had about your ability to change.

The spark for a successful lifestyle change must come from within. External factors may play a role in pushing you to action, but true commitment can come only from inside you.

Ask yourself, "Do I know how to change?" Many people skip vital steps in their rush to see results, making the process of change almost impossible. You may be thinking, "Now there's a *way* to change?" There always was. But until recently, people who successfully altered their lifestyles did so without the benefit of a proven model for change. They went through a process of trial and error until they finally got it right. Not until James Prochaska and two of his colleagues, John Norcross and Carlo DiClemente, all professors of psychology, developed the Transtheoretical Approach for Change did people understand that the process of change involved more than just taking action (beginning an exercise program).

This approach is now the standard for many behavioral-change programs today. It addresses the phases that lead up to taking action, then identifies the phases that exist after action is taken. Too often in the past action has been equated with change. Action is not change but merely *part of the process* of change.

Reading this book is one part of the process that will help you to change successfully.

The Transtheoretical Approach for Change

According to the Transtheoretical Approach, there are six stages to change:

- Precontemplation

- Contemplation

- Preparation

- Action

- Maintenance

- Termination

The stage most often missed is Preparation. People often jump from Contemplation into Action, making the Maintenance stage (continuation of proper eating habits and exercise) unsustainable. The Termination stage, in which the undesirable behaviours such as eating improperly and not exercising are ended, cannot be permanent without the successful completion of the previous stages.

Within these six stages of change there are nine processes that you can use to help you move from one stage of change to the next. These processes are Consciousness-Raising, Social Liberation, Emotional Arousal, Self-Evaluation, Commitment, Countering, Environmental Control, Reward, and

Helping Relationships. Don't let the names of the processes throw you off. As we look at the stages of change, you will see how each one of these processes can be translated into a valuable tool to make change possible. It is important to use the proper process tools for each different stage of change. While all of the tools can be used in more than one stage, as you change you will gradually switch the tools you are using, to continue your journey and make your changes permanent.

Stage One: *Precontemplation*

*P*recontemplation could be referred to as the invisible stage, because a person in this stage does not seem to be changing at all. Precontemplators might not even acknowledge that they have a problem or have any intention of changing. They will usually resist all suggestions from loved ones that they should alter their lifestyles. Precontemplators will often try to justify their lifestyles — saying that they have no time or listing other barriers — or will change the subject. Those who try to push Precontemplators into action will have a hard time getting them to change a problem they won't even acknowledge.

Precontemplators can also be people who have tried unsuccessfully in the past to change their unhealthy behaviours. Their lack of success is probably due to their having skipped the Contemplation and Preparation stages of change, moving straight into the Action stage.

Do you think you are in the Precontemplation stage? If you bought this book, you are probably in one of the later stages. Do you intend to change your eating habits or to start exercising in the next six months? If your answer is no, you are in the Precontemplation stage.

If you have a friend or loved one who is in the Precontemplation stage, you can help them move into the Contemplation stage by using the process tools of Consciousness-Raising and Social Liberation.

Consciousness-Raising involves becoming aware of your eating and exercise habits and trying to identify why you do not want to change. Is your lifestyle a choice or has it just evolved? If it was not a conscious choice, why are you not changing your unhealthy habits? The more information you can accumulate about why you haven't changed and how you defend your inability to act, the more likely it is that you will be able to move to the next stage of change. In other words, you must be able to identify the means you use to justify your current lifestyle. We will discuss in detail how to identify your barriers and obstacles — and the excuses you use — in the next chapter.

There are several strategies you can employ to help you increase your awareness and understanding of why you need to change:

- Read a book about people who have changed their eating or exercise habits.
- Subscribe to a health-and-fitness magazine.
- Watch a television show relating to exercise and eating habits.
- Talk to friends or family members who have made lifestyle changes about the process they went through.
- Have a complete medical examination to get a neutral opinion on the state of your health and the consequences of your lifestyle choices.

Social Liberation is the support, information, and encouragement offered by our social institutions to people with behaviours they want to change. In the last ten years, smoking has become socially unacceptable. Society no longer accepts the choice to smoke and has placed limits on where smokers can indulge their addiction. At the same time, though, stop-smoking programs and public-health information on the dangers of tobacco have become available. Many workplaces now offer on-site fitness facilities to encourage their employees to exercise. The self-help movement offers individuals who may feel they are the only person with a particular problem the opportunity to talk and learn from others who share the same goals. Here are some strategies you can use to reinforce the desire to change through the process of Social Liberation:

- Start going to restaurants that offer a healthy-heart menu (low-fat meal choices).
- Take a low-fat-cooking class.

- Attend a lecture or workshop on how to begin an exercise program.
- Investigate whether your (or your spouse's) workplace offers an on-site fitness facility or provides funding for you to join an outside facility.

The difficulty you may encounter when trying to help Precontemplators is the refusal to acknowledge lifestyle problems. Do not try to push a Precontemplator into taking action. Do be supportive and persistent in offering encouragement. You will require a lot of patience, but eventually your efforts will pay off. The worst thing you can do to people in the Precontemplation stage is to give up, enabling them to continue unhealthy habits and reinforcing the feeling that change is not necessary.

Stage Two: *Contemplation*

*Y*ou have acknowledged that you want to start exercising or change your eating habits because you aren't satisfied with your present lifestyle. You have not picked a date to start but you know that you will change your bad habits — someday. Yet, when it's time to actually start, you always find a good reason not to. The Contemplation stage feels comfortable because you have made a vague commitment to change sometime in the future. However, you never seem to find the time, energy, or motivation to start because the demands of everyday life constantly get in the way. You are aware of the problem but do not focus on a solution. This is the stage most of us live in from day to day.

If you bought this book to learn more about how you can change your eating habits or start exercising, and you have not yet acted, you are in the Contemplation stage. The problem you may have is that you know you want to change, yet you are still resisting, hanging on to a lifestyle that is familiar, safe, and comfortable.

In the Contemplation stage, you should use the process tools of Emotional Arousal and Self-Evaluation.

Emotions play a powerful role in our lives. They colour our thinking when we make decisions and influence what those decisions will be. Emotions can move us forward or hold us back. You can learn how to use your emotions to create the spark of inspiration that will propel you from Contemplation to Preparation. Here are some helpful strategies for *Emotional Arousal*:

- Seek out movies, television specials, or old news stories about people who have struggled with a weight problem or poor eating habits.
- Create a visual image that puts your food choices in perspective. For example, if you love your mashed potatoes smothered in gravy, imagine placing them in a blender and liquefying them. Picture pouring the resulting "soup" into a see-through container and watching the fat rise to the surface. Imagine yourself eating this, grease and all.
- Picture yourself in three, five, and ten years without having changed your eating or exercise habits. Imagine how you will feel, how you will look, and how your health and appearance will affect the people around you.
- Take out some old clothes that you would like to fit into again. Put them on and look at yourself in the mirror.
- Imagine that the worst has happened: your current lifestyle choices have led you to an early death from heart disease. Write a letter to your spouse and children, explaining why and how you died, and trying to make amends for all that you have missed doing with them.

With *Self-Evaluation* you take a real look at yourself, your eating habits, and the lack of exercise in your life. First focus on the present and evaluate how your current lifestyle makes you feel. Would your life be better if you changed your habits? Can you say that you are happy with the way you feel about yourself and your unhealthy behaviours? What would you have to give up to change your lifestyle? Next, think of how your life would be if you made these changes. Be realistic in your views. Evaluate how you would feel if you led a healthier life. Successful Self-Evaluation will cause you to really think about your lifestyle, and you will conclude that you could have a better quality of life if you changed your exercise or eating habits.

Here are some strategies to help you use Self-Evaluation as a tool to move you beyond Contemplation:

- Pause before you eat an unhealthy snack and ask yourself if it's really what you want or if you are eating because you are feeling stressed or unhappy. Or have you simply formed a habit of eating a certain food at a certain time?
- Write out the pros and cons of changing your lifestyle. Make a list for yourself, then make a second list of how these changes would affect the people around you. How would your spouse and children benefit or lose by your changes?
- Picture yourself before and after you have changed. Write down words to describe how you feel now and how you would feel afterwards.

If you have recognized that you are in either the Precontemplation or the Contemplation stage, take the time to use the tools and strategies described; until you do, do not continue to read the rest of the book. Towards the end of the Contemplation stage, you will notice that you are focusing on possible solutions rather than on your unhealthy habits, and you will begin to think about the future instead of dwelling on the past. You should then continue with the rest of this chapter, use the tools in the Preparation stage, and then read the rest of the book before you act.

Stage Three: *Preparation*

*I*f you think about it, you will realize that most of your greatest accomplishments have been the result of hard work, planning, and preparation. Many successful people live by the "4P Rule": "Poor planning leads to pretty poor results." But the Preparation stage is the most often overlooked stage of change. Many people go through the Precontemplation to the Contemplation stage and then take action. But those who have been successful at permanently changing their eating and exercise habits have taken the time to plan exactly how they were going to accomplish their goals.

During the Preparation stage you need to look over all the options that are available and decide which are best suited to your circumstances and temperament. For example, is it best to join a fitness facility because you want to be around other people who have similar goals, to invest in a piece of home exercise equipment, or to take long walks? If you decide to join a fitness facility, when would you exercise, and what type of exercise do you think you would enjoy the most? If you are going to take long walks, where and when will you go? Alone or with a buddy? If you are going to change your eating habits, which foods will you cut out, which ones will you modify, and how will you stay on track?

These are questions that someone in the Preparation phase should resolve by means of a detailed plan. In this stage, you will no longer focus on getting information about the consequences of lack of exercise and poor eating habits but rather on how you can change your current habits. Although you may have some lingering doubts about your ability to change, you are more confident that you are making the right decision.

Many people short-circuit the Preparation phase — which should last up to a month — because they do not take adequate time to gather all the information about their alternatives. If they want to start exercising, for example, they may buy an exercise video without asking themselves whether they need the stimulation and motivation of exercising with other people at a fitness facility. Explore all your options concerning where and when you will exercise, and what exercise you will do. The same goes for changing your eating habits.

Consciousness-Raising, Social Liberation, Emotional Arousal, and Self-Evaluation carry over into the Preparation stage. A new process tool also comes into play: Commitment.

Do not confuse Commitment with words like "willpower" and "determination." *Commitment* to your new lifestyle is a tool that you will use on a day-to-day basis. When you get married, you commit yourself to the person you are marrying. Do you vow to use "willpower" or "determination" to keep your marriage together? Of course not! You are committed to making your marriage work because you are confident about the choice you have made.

The same can be said about your decision to lead a healthier lifestyle. When you are confident you are making the right choice, your commitment to making the changes increases. Here are some useful tools you can use to reinforce your commitment and move on to the Action stage:

- Take a good look at the decision you have made to change your lifestyle. Ask yourself if you feel committed to these changes.
- Look at your day-to-day schedule. Implementing exercise and healthier eating habits will require your time. Since there are only so many hours in a day, ask yourself what you are willing to put aside to make time for your new activities.
- Set a specific date to start exercising. Make sure that it is no longer than a month away.
- Buy anything you will need, including new running shoes and exercise apparel.
- Buy a piece of home exercise equipment or take out a fitness club membership for next month.
- Tell people around you the date you plan to start exercising and changing your diet.

Stage Four: *Action*

*T*he Action stage requires the most time and energy, both physical and mental. Although most people feel they have already changed when they reach the Action stage, in reality they are still in the process of changing.

This phase can be filled with mixed emotions: you will be excited as you experience feelings of success after completing a workout; and you will feel frustrated by the people and events around you that compete for your time and energy. The following four process tools can help you during the Action phase: Countering, Environmental Control, Reward, and Helping Relationships.

Countering is the act of substituting one act or behaviour for another. For example: you have had a horrible day at work and come home tired and stressed. You eat a healthy supper and then eye a bag of potato chips in the cupboard. Right away you start to think about sinking down on the couch and devouring the whole bag. Instead, however, you decide to take a walk. You have countered an unhealthy behaviour with a healthy behaviour.

If you have already exercised that day, you can substitute another activity such as lighting some candles in the bathroom and taking a warm relaxing bath, or doing some light gardening. Choose a healthy activity that you enjoy and that helps you relax. Once you have finished the countering activity, you will find that your momentary cravings have passed.

Environmental Control means avoiding situations that undermine your positive actions. No matter how committed you are to exercising and eating properly, it will be difficult to sustain that commitment if you are constantly in an environment where you are tempted to revert to your former lifestyle. Lack of Environmental Control is like buying groceries while you are hungry: everything appeals to you and the urge to buy unhealthy food wins out over your commitment. Do not allow yourself to be put in situations where you know you will be tempted to eat all the wrong foods or skip a scheduled workout. To increase your chances, exercise control over your own environment. Remove junk food from your home. Do not schedule a lunch with friends a couple of hours before you are supposed to exercise. By consciously controlling your environment, you can increase your chances of keeping the commitment you have made to live a healthier life.

Reward is the process by which we acknowledge our own need for positive reinforcement. Too often we berate ourselves when we have a bad day. If we eat something we wanted to avoid, or skip a workout, we can be our own worst enemies. Yet, when we are doing well, we often fail to reward ourselves. Set up your own series of rewards — such as going to a movie that you want to see or buying a new accessory that you want — on a weekly basis. Rewards do not have to be expensive. You can reward yourself by soaking in the tub while listening to classical music or by allowing yourself an extra half hour to pursue a hobby you enjoy. Pick rewards that have special meaning to you.

Another way to reward yourself is to put two dollars away in a jar — or whatever you can afford — each week that you continue with your new healthy habits. This money can go towards a vacation you have always wanted to take, your children's education, or your favourite charity. The last suggestion provides you with the satisfaction of doing something to improve the lives of others while you work to improve your own — the feeling that you get from helping someone else is a great source of motivation.

Helping Relationships provides the social context that boosts motivation. While it is important to have the help and support of others through all the stages of change, it becomes vital during the Action stage. Find an exercise partner — having someone to walk with can be fun as well as motivational. Start eating properly with someone who has also made a commitment to a healthier lifestyle. You might find an "exercise partner" on the Internet with whom you can share your frustrations and triumphs while gaining and giving support.

The following strategies will help you move through the Action stage into the Maintenance stage:

- Write down possible activities to use as a substitute for urges to eat junk food.
- Make a list of the types of situations or environments that will tempt you to overeat or skip a scheduled workout.
- Develop strategies to help you change or avoid these situations.
- Develop a reward system.
- Identify people who can help and support you.

Stage Five: *Maintenance*

*Y*ou have no doubt heard stories about people who lost a lot of weight only to put it all back on months or years later. They simply could not maintain the healthier lifestyle they had adopted. Restrictive diets, unrealistic goals, external factors that cause emotional upheaval, and social situations that cause temptation can lead us back to our old behaviours. We tend to forget how bad we felt before we started to exercise and eat properly. The lack of energy and self-confidence and the feelings of stress fade from our memories. Apathy sets in and old behaviours resurface.

Some of you may view action as your only goal; once you have taken action, your commitment starts to fade — along with any results you have realized. Other priorities start gaining precedence and before you know it, you have abandoned your plans to change. This shifting of priorities provides you with a "way out" to justify your unconscious decision to quit: "My job got too hectic" or "My children got the flu."

The Maintenance stage requires intense patience and perseverance. Because this stage can last for many months — or even years — you remain at risk for returning to your former unhealthy behaviours. Along the way, you will have days when your new lifestyle seems easy to maintain, and days when you give in to temptation. Even when you have reached your weight-loss or fitness goal, you have not reached your greater goal of staying fit forever.

Lapses are common among people who are trying to change. To expect yourself to have a perfect track record would be unrealistic and would damage your belief that you can change. We will discuss how to handle lapses and prevent relapses in Chapter Eight. The key to maintenance is long-term commitment applied on a day-to-day basis, and maintenance should be a part of your overall goals.

The processes which are most useful during the Maintenance stage are Commitment, Reward, Countering, Environment Control, and Helping Relationships.

Again, the Maintenance stage can last for months or for years and will end when you reach the Termination stage.

Stage Six: *Termination*

*A*ll of you who are trying to change your lifestyles have the same goal: to instill new healthier habits into your lives while eliminating unhealthy habits. You will know you have reached the Termination stage when you no longer feel tempted to resume your old unhealthy behaviours. Situations that would have been a problem in the past no longer threaten you, and you do not have to struggle on a day-to-day basis to continue exercising and eating properly. You have terminated your former unhealthy habits and have permanently substituted exercise and eating properly as vital components in your life.

Case Study *Life's Lessons*

After her fourth child was born, at the of age thirty-five Beth decided that she wanted to lose some weight. She went on a successful diet but she couldn't imagine sustaining it for longer than a couple of months. She cooked regular meals for her family and acknowledged that it was a constant temptation to eat what her family was eating — which she often did. A self-proclaimed yo-yo dieter, Beth lost and regained weight repeatedly. She constantly bounced between the Contemplation stage and the Action stage.

By age forty Beth was divorced from her husband and was forced to support four school-age children. She had two years of college under her belt, and knew she would have to go back to school to get a degree. She decided that she wanted to become a social worker. But when she investigated various schools, she learned she would be unable to transfer most of her early college credits towards obtaining her degree. Convinced that her decision was still the right one for herself and her family, she enrolled in the first year of a university social-work program. Before Beth could begin school, she had to plan how she was going to take care of four children, work part-time, attend university, and find the time to study. Beth had to re-organize her entire life — thoroughly plan her schedule in advance, identify potential scheduling problems, and prioritize all aspects of her life — if she was going make it to graduation *and* balance the needs of her family.

Beth decided to work three days a week and go to school two days a week. She organized her time so that she would be home when the children finished school. She helped with homework, cooked supper, and did laundry. Her children knew that every night at 8:00 was Mom's time to study. Beth told them how important it was that she have this time and her children supported her. It wasn't easy, but Beth went on to obtain her degree and began her career.

At age fifty-five Beth started to realize that she had to make some changes. She was the director of a program for victims of violent crime and her job was very stressful. She also wanted to reduce her weight. Her children were adults with successful careers and families of their own. They had always been physically active, and now she thought about exercising herself. She made a decision to learn more about exercise and how to eat a healthier diet. Beth had already experienced the value of preparation in successful change when she decided to go back to school. She now looked at different types of exercise and what her alternatives were. She sought out information about less restrictive diets. Beth then used the organizational skills she had learned by going to school, working, and raising four children and applied them to her decision to implement lifestyle changes. Beth moved quickly from Precontemplation to Contemplation to Preparation to Action.

Ten years later, at age sixty-five, Beth runs three to four miles a day, three days a week. She prefers to run outside, but when the weather is bad she goes to a fitness centre. Beth also attends aquafitness classes four or five days a week. She maintains her eating habits and exercise by foreseeing daily obstacles and developing alternative strategies. She has reached her goals and says that it is no longer a struggle to exercise and eat properly. She has reached the Termination stage of change. Beth has advice for people thinking about making changes in their lives: "You have to get all the information available about the changes that you want to make and be committed to reaching your goals. You have to make the time and prioritize the things that are most important to you."

Ten Key Steps to Success

Change can be wonderful and exciting, but when we are not ready to change it can also be frustrating and frightening. Many of you who have tried before to exercise and eat properly but reverted to your old behaviours can recognize where you had problems and learn to correct them. Remember that any past attempts to exercise and eat properly were not failures but practice. You have learned from your prior attempts what does not work for you. You now have more information and more insight about the process of change, and can make it work for you.

1 Read about all the stages of change and decide which one you are in.

2 Understand that people in the Precontemplation stage are in denial and need the help of others.

3 Seek out information during the Contemplation stage about the benefits of eating properly and exercising.

4 Start reading about how to cook tasty low-fat meals and how to safely begin an exercise program.

5 Acknowledge that there will never be a "perfect time" to start exercising and eating better.

6 Start focusing on possible solutions to your problems and start developing alternatives to your current behaviours.

7 Read the rest of this book and complete the questionnaires before you act, so you are thoroughly prepared to begin.

8 Realize that action is only one part of change.

9 Decide how you will reward yourself for exercising and eating properly on a weekly basis. Base your rewards on successfully keeping all your scheduled workouts and eating properly rather than on physical results.

10 Make maintenance a part of your ongoing goals.

Barriers, Obstacles, or Excuses?

$\mathcal{W}$e all have reasons why we cannot exercise. Some are legitimate but most are not. No rationalization can erase the fact that being overweight is a known risk factor for diabetes, heart disease, high blood pressure, arthritis, and some forms of cancer, or that exercising decreases the effects of osteoporosis, and can greatly improve our quality of life as we age.

If we know the consequences of not exercising and not eating properly, why do we persist in these bad habits? Do you know anyone who has openly admitted that he wants to shorten his life span and die of a disease he could have prevented? Of course not! Just talk to people who have suffered preventable heart attacks and they will tell you they wish they had chosen a healthier lifestyle. Until we experience serious health problems, we imagine we are immune. When they happen, we react with shock and disbelief, blaming fate or believing that our bodies have betrayed us. We ignore the role our own behaviours played, relieving ourselves of any responsibility.

Our reasons for not taking care of ourselves fall into three categories: barriers, obstacles, and excuses.

A *barrier* is an unpreventable event or circumstance that hinders our plans or actions. For example, when you are on your way to the gym, your car breaks down. By the time you arrange for a tow truck and get a ride home, you have missed the fitness class you wanted to go to and are feeling too frustrated and tired to attend a later one.

An *obstacle* is a foreseeable event or circumstance that impedes our plans or actions. For example, your spouse travels for work every third week and your increased responsibilities at home, and the need to get a babysitter if you go out, make exercising too difficult.

An *excuse* is an event or circumstance, foreseeable or unforeseeable, that with planning could be overcome. One of the classic excuses is not having "enough time."

When we identify all our barriers and obstacles we see how many are actually excuses. Sometimes we expend more energy justifying our failure to do what we know we should than we would have if we had just done it. Think about times you have had to write a report for work or a term paper. You put it off until the very last minute, but once you got started, you realized the project was not as difficult as you thought it would be. When you finished you felt relieved and proud of what you had done. Just like the term paper or work report, our bodies have deadlines. Give yourself the chance to choose your own deadline to start eating properly and exercising, rather than having it forced on you by your doctor or by catastrophic illness.

By now you have identified time in your schedule to exercise two to three times per week, blocked out a time to plan in advance what you are going to eat for a week, and allotted the time to prepare it. You have also made a made a contract with yourself to follow through with your decision to lead a healthy lifestyle.

It is now time to list any event or circumstance that might hinder your efforts to honour your contract and stop you from starting or sticking with your healthy-lifestyle program. These reasons may include working overtime, appointments for you or another family member, or social obligations. On the following chart write down anything that might postpone your getting started, make you skip a workout, or make a dash by the drive-through window at your favourite fast-food restaurant.

What Is Stopping Me?

	Reason	Barrier	Obstacle	Excuse
1				
2				
3				
4				
5				
6				
7				
8				
9				
10				

Look over your reasons carefully and think about each one. Can you tell whether a reason is a barrier, an obstacle, or an excuse? When you can logically determine what each one of your roadblocks is, you can develop different strategies to overcome all of them.

If you were driving a car and came to a roadblock, would you try to drive through it? If you couldn't drive through it, would you go back to where you began, or follow the detour signs to your final destination? A detour may take time and energy, but it will get you to your destination a lot faster than going back to where you started.

Identifying Personal Barriers

$\mathcal{A}$ barrier is an unpreventable event or circumstance that hinders your plans or actions. For example, you know that in the next three weeks work is going to be hectic and you will have to stay late some evenings, missing some fitness classes. Working late when needed is an assumed condition of your job and cannot be changed. This is a barrier.

Look at your list of reasons again. Can you better identify which of your reasons are barriers? Put a check mark in the barrier column beside each one.

Foreseeing Obstacles

Obstacles are hindering events or circumstances that you *can* prevent or remove. When your days are full, with work, appointments, and family obligations, it may be difficult to see how you can fit everything in. But you have to remember that although your days are full, you *can* rearrange your schedule to make more efficient use of the time you do have. For instance, find ways to increase your productivity at work so you do not have to bring work home or work late. If you have to drive your children to swimming practice, exercise in the same facility while they swim, or start a car pool with other parents to give yourself time to prepare a nutritious dinner.

Look again at your list of reasons to see which are obstacles, and place a check mark in the obstacle column beside each one.

Some obstacles pop up at the last minute. Although these are unexpected at the time, you can usually predict that an event or circumstance might occasionally happen and make provisions for them. For example, what can you do if your usual babysitter cannot come? What can you do if you unexpectedly have to work late? It is inevitable that these events will happen sooner or later, but most of us make the mistake of not planning for them.

Go back to your list of reasons and add any obstacles you did not think of before. Place a check mark beside them in the obstacle column.

If you still have reasons that have not been categorized, they are probably excuses. Ask yourself, "Is this something that I can change or, if not, is it something that I can work around by rearranging other variables?"

When you plan for barriers and obstacles you stand a much better chance of having the time to reach your goals. You won't get sidetracked and become frustrated that you cannot stick to your lifestyle changes. Many of us get caught up in the day-to-day demands on our time and ignore the long-term effects our schedules are having on our health. We all have the power to change our schedules, just as we all have the right to devote an hour each day to taking care of ourselves.

Your obstacles and barriers will change from day to day, month to month, and year to year. It is important to identify your barriers and obstacles on a monthly basis. Try to pick a specific day — say, the first of each month — to go through your day planner and note new barriers or obstacles for that month.

Developing Strategies That Work

 O ne of the biggest challenges you will have to face when trying to reach your goal of changing your lifestyle is to keep from falling back into old behaviours. Most people have foods that they use to comfort or reward themselves; exercise, in the beginning, can cause you discomfort. Do not let the temptation of comforting food or a rest for your aching muscles deter you from your goals.

When an event forces you to miss a scheduled workout, it is easy to say, "I will do it tomorrow." The next day, because you have not scheduled exercise into your day, it may be hard to find the time. "Oh well, I am supposed to work out tomorrow anyway, so I'll forget about it for today," is the standard excuse. What happens if something comes up again the next day? This is how many people fall into the cycle of failure. They begin to miss scheduled workouts and never see any results because they have not been able to exercise consistently. They become demotivated and fall back into their negative patterns.

One way to prevent relapsing into old behaviours is to develop strategies that counteract your personal barriers and obstacles. These strategies will help you stay on track — and because you will have planned for a particular problem in advance, less conscious effort on your part will be needed to follow through with your intentions.

Let's look at someone we will call Anne. Anne works in the banking industry and is the mother of two school-age children. Her husband, Tom, is a district manager of a retail chain of stores. She lists the following reasons for why she cannot start or stick with her lifestyle changes: 1. My work schedule varies depending on the workload; 2. My husband sometimes has to work late; 3. I am sometimes hungry after work and need to snack on whatever is handy while preparing dinner.

Most people have a lot more than three barriers and obstacles, but the three reasons listed above were enough to prevent Anne from losing the pounds she had been trying to shed for five years.

The next step to developing strategies that work is to determine how your barriers and obstacles influence your actions.

Anne placed her work schedule in the barrier column. She felt she could do nothing about her varying workload, which made it impossible for her to regularly attend her fitness class. Anne placed her next two reasons in the obstacle category.

Anne needed to think more about her barriers and obstacles and come up with strategies she felt comfortable with should these situations occur. Look at the following Lifestyle Planning Worksheet and see how Anne decided that she could overcome her personal barriers and obstacles.

Anne's Lifestyle Planning Worksheet

Barriers

1. *My work schedule varies depending on my workload.*

   Result: *I will miss some scheduled workouts.*

Strategy A: *I will ask if I can complete some work at home.*

Strategy B: *I will find out whether there is a fitness class I can attend on my lunch hour or after my children are in bed.*

Strategy C: *I will purchase a stationary bike or treadmill so I can do the cardiovascular part of my workouts at home when this happens.*

Obstacles

1. *My husband sometimes has to work late and I have to be at home to take care of the children.*

   Result: *I will miss the fitness class I like to go to.*

Strategy A: *I will ask my daytime sitter if she is available to stay late when this happens.*

Strategy B: *I will develop a list of three babysitters that can come on short notice.*

Strategy C: *I will work out on my treadmill or exercise bike after my children have gone to bed.*

2. *I am hungry when I get home from work and pick at foods while I am preparing dinner.*

      Result: *I eat about five cookies while I am preparing supper and feel guilty after I have eaten them.*

      Strategy A: *I will prepare and bring a healthy snack that I will eat mid-afternoon.*

      Strategy B: *I will prepare some healthy snacks and put them in the refrigerator so they are handy when I get home.*

      Strategy C: *I will plan what the family is going to eat, and whenever possible ask the babysitter to place it in the oven so that supper is nearly ready when I get home.*

It is one thing to have a plan and another to put that plan into action. In Anne's case, she must take several steps to ensure that her strategies are successful. Anne must create a list of what she needs to do and apply time frames for completing everything on her list. This task can be done using the Lifestyle Planning Checklist:

Anne's Lifestyle Planning Checklist

To Do	Time frame	Done (✓)
1. Ask my boss if I can take work home.	Tomorrow	
2. Purchase a stationary bike or treadmill.	This weekend	
3. Ask my sitter if she can stay late if needed.	Tomorrow	
4. Bring a snack to work each day.	Tomorrow	
5. Put a healthy snack in the fridge for tomorrow.	Tonight	✓
6. Get the telephone numbers of three sitters for emergencies.	By next week	
7. Start planning next week's meals.	By Sunday	

List your own barriers and obstacles on the following chart. Then write down three strategies that will help you to overcome each one.

Lifestyle Planning Worksheet – Barriers

1. ....

    Result: ....

                    ....

Strategy A: ....

Strategy B: ....

Strategy C: ....

                    ....

2. ....

    Result: ....

                    ....

Strategy A: ....

Strategy B: ....

Strategy C: ....

                    ....

3. ....

    Result: ....

                    ....

Strategy A: ....

Strategy B: ....

Strategy C: ....

                    ....

4. ....

    Result: ....

                    ....

Strategy A: ....

Strategy B: ....

Strategy C: ....

                    ....

Lifestyle Planning Worksheet – <u>Obstacles</u>

1. ....

    Result: ....

  Strategy A: ....

  Strategy B: ....

  Strategy C: ....

2. ....

    Result: ....

  Strategy A: ....

  Strategy B: ....

  Strategy C: ....

3. ....

    Result: ....

  Strategy A: ....

  Strategy B: ....

  Strategy C: ....

4. ....

    Result: ....

  Strategy A: ....

  Strategy B: ....

  Strategy C: ....

Examine your strategies and list the steps you will need to take on the Lifestyle Planning Checklist, along with an appropriate time frame:

Lifestyle Planning Checklist

	To Do	Time frame	Done (✓)
1			
2			
3			
4			
5			
6			
7			
8			
9			
10			

Case Study *Excuses, Excuses*

Patricia is a thirty-nine-year-old homemaker and the mother of two children. Her friend, Cindy, also thirty-nine, has lost twenty-two pounds and has kept them off for two years. Patricia and Cindy meet up at a neighbourhood barbecue. Cindy overhears Patricia joking with some of the other women about losing weight. Patricia says that four years ago she had wanted to lose five pounds but had not found the time to exercise. These five pounds had over time turned into twenty pounds. "I'm either going to have to start a diet, or get pregnant to justify this weight. Guess I'll get pregnant . . . it's easier," she jests. Everyone laughs.

As people drift away, Cindy watches her friend's expression grow sad as she stares at the cheeseburger and potato chips on her paper plate. Cindy goes over and chats for a few minutes before she brings up Patricia's comment: "That was pretty funny. I assume that you're not going to get pregnant again — " she laughs — "so when are you going to start exercising?"

"Oh," Patricia says, "I can't start now. It isn't a good time."

"Why not?" Cindy asks.

"Well, Brian is travelling a lot for work and I have to take care of the kids. There just isn't enough time during the day."

"What about at night? You could get a babysitter," Cindy suggests.

"I have to bathe the kids and I wouldn't feel comfortable with a babysitter doing it. The boys won't let anyone but me bathe them, anyway."

"How old are the boys now?" Cindy asks, already knowing the answer.

"Eight and ten." Patricia smiles.

"Maybe they could bathe themselves or have their baths before the babysitter gets there."

"I suppose they could do that, but I can't justify buying another piece of exercise equipment. My last exercise bike sat in the basement until I finally sold it."

"Why don't you just go for a walk? You could take your dog and you wouldn't have to buy anything new."

"Well, with the boys' hockey, music lessons, and everything else I couldn't walk three to four times a week," Patricia fires back, feeling somewhat irked by Cindy's persistence.

"How many times *could* you walk?" Cindy asks.

"Twice, maybe."

"Why don't you make that your goal — to walk two times a week. That way, if you get an extra day in, it will be a bonus, rather than trying for three to four times, knowing it will be almost impossible to do."

"I guess I could do that," Patricia admits, looking away.

"OK, so what is stopping you?" Cindy asks.

"I guess just me. If I really wanted to, I could make the time to exercise. I just never thought beyond all the reasons why I couldn't," Patricia says ruefully.

Patricia has several reasons why she cannot find the time to exercise, but none are barriers or obstacles that she could not overcome if she committed herself to developing strategies to ensure success.

Ten Key Steps to Success

*E*veryone has reasons why they cannot exercise and eat properly. These reasons cause most people to operate on autopilot: "I can't . . . I don't have enough time . . . my work schedule makes exercise impossible." When you identify each reason and analyze it individually, you take an important step towards controlling your health, happiness, and well-being. Control your life; don't let your life control you.

1   Identify and write down all your reasons for not starting or not persisting with an exercise program and proper eating habits.

2   Classify your reasons as barriers or obstacles.

3   Decide how your barriers and obstacles will affect the lifestyle changes you wish to make.

4   Come up with several strategies to deal with each barrier and obstacle.

5   Examine your strategies to determine which are viable.

6   Write down the two or three best strategies for overcoming each of your barriers and obstacles.

7   List the steps you need to take to make your strategies for workable actions and apply time frames to each step.

8   Review your barriers and obstacles at the beginning of each month.

9   Identify any new barriers and obstacles.

10   Create new strategies and a checklist for your changing barriers and obstacles, as needed.

4

Goal Setting
for Success

$\mathcal{T}$oo often people set unreachable goals for themselves: not only can the actual goal be unrealistic but also the time frame placed on reaching it. Many people do not realize that it took months, maybe even years, of inactivity and poor eating habits for them to reach their current physical condition. If it took that long to get out of shape, does it make sense to allow less time to get fit again?

Everyone wants instant gratification and instant results. Want to lose twenty pounds in a month? Drink a diet milkshake or pop a pill that will suppress your appetite. But once you stop taking that pill, the weight is sure to come back and you will be more discouraged than ever. The key to reaching your goals and staying there is to take your time and teach yourself to change the behaviours that made you gain weight or become unfit.

Many of you probably already have specific goals in mind. Is your goal truly the end result you are looking for, or is it rather a means to get to an underlying goal? Let's take a look at the different types of goals and how they can affect your overall view of what you want to achieve.

Surface Goals and Underlying Goals

$\mathcal{O}$ne type of goal is a *surface goal* — something we think we must achieve (for example, losing ten pounds) in order to gain something else. That something else is our *underlying goal* — usually a feeling or a state of mind, such as pride in our appearance or a sense of well-being about our health. We must identify and understand our underlying goals so that we know where the journey of self-change is taking us, and when we have completed it.

Say you decide you want to lose ten pounds because your clothes are all starting to feel tight. You set your goal of losing ten pounds and apply a realistic time frame of three months. You reach your goal within that time frame and for the first two weeks afterwards you feel great. During the third week, however, you start to feel unsatisfied but cannot figure out why: your surface goal — losing ten pounds — was not your underlying goal, which was to feel healthy and in control.

We all have underlying goals that we have not identified. If your surface goal does not help you achieve your underlying goal, you will have a hard time motivating yourself to exercise and eat properly on a day-to-day basis.

Bob, a forty-six-year-old executive, decided to hire a personal trainer to help him lose fifteen pounds after his wife repeatedly commented on his weight. He scheduled a meeting with the trainer to discuss his goals and the cost:

"Hello Bob. My name is Steven. I'm the trainer who spoke to you on the telephone. It is nice to meet you."

"Hi, Steven," Bob said, sitting down across from Steven.

"Bob, why are you considering hiring a personal fitness trainer?"

"My wife thinks I need to lose about fifteen pounds."

"And what do you think, Bob?"

"I guess I could lose some weight, but what I would really like to do is increase my energy level."

"How would having more energy affect your day-to-day life?" Steven asked.

"If I had more energy I might start playing racquetball again. I enjoyed it. There is a group from work that still plays."

"Are these people co-workers or friends? Do you socialize with them outside racquetball?"

"They're both, but I don't see them outside work anymore," Bob replied.

Steven recapped what he thought Bob's goals were. "You want to lose approximately fifteen pounds and get in better physical condition so you can increase your energy level and start playing racquetball with your friends."

"That about covers it," Bob smiled. Bob inquired about the fee, filled out a health history, and set up a series of training appointments with Steven. While driving home Bob thought about how good it would be to get back into his old routine. He always enjoyed the verbal sparring that went on during the games and the tournaments that they set up once in a while. "I wonder if Jim is still beating the pants off everyone. I was the only one who could really make him run," he recalled.

Bob's surface goal was to lose fifteen pounds. His underlying goal was to be part of his group of friends again. He felt lonely and alienated from his old crowd. Losing weight was just a means to an end. If Steven had not asked Bob how he thought having more energy would affect his day-to-day routine, Bob might not have realized that he wanted to play racquetball and, in turn, renew his old friendships. Even if Bob had lost his fifteen pounds he would not have satisfied his emotional needs, and he would probably have regained the weight within a few months.

What is your underlying reason for wanting to change your lifestyle? If your goal is to lose weight, ask yourself, "Why do I want to lose weight?" If your goal is to increase your strength, ask yourself why. Insert your goal into the following statement and complete the sentence.

I want to ....

because ....

The first part of the sentence is your surface goal and the second part is your underlying goal. You may have to fill in the sentence more than once to get at your true goal, so use a pencil.

Once you understand what your underlying goal is, you have uncovered your true motivation. If you can acknowledge what is driving you to make changes in your life, you'll have a much better chance of reaching both your surface and underlying goals.

Intrinsic and Extrinsic Goals

*I*n an informal survey of more than three hundred personal trainers in the United States and Canada, 78 percent responded that one of the main reasons clients wanted to start an exercise program was to lose weight. The average weight loss desired was between fifteen and twenty pounds. While these trainers believed that weight loss was their clients' only goal, it is usually only a surface goal.

Any goal that can be measured by an external mechanism is an ***extrinsic goal***. Losing weight, increasing your muscular strength and endurance, and improving your cardiovascular system or flexibility are all examples of goals that can be measured by a conventional fitness appraisal.

Intrinsic goals, on the other hand, are goals whose achievement only you can measure. An increase in energy, decreased stress, and a better quality of sleep are all examples of intrinsic goals. Intrinsic goals differ from underlying goals because they involve physical change, not emotional change. It is important to understand that surface goals are extrinsic goals but that underlying goals differ from intrinsic goals. All these types of goals can overlap; achieving one type will affect your ability to achieve another.

People reach their goals at different speeds. How long it will take you to reach your surface goals depends on heredity, current fitness level, and health restrictions. Although there are averages for weight loss and gains in muscular strength and endurance, you must remember what "average" means. Some people must necessarily fall into the high and low ranges to create an average. If you fall into the low range, it becomes even more important to set goals that you will reach in a short period: when you reach that first goal, you will be motivated to continue in order to see further results.

Setting intrinsic goals plays an important role in helping you achieve other types of goals. Most people will reach an intrinsic goal before they reach a surface goal. Take Bob, for instance. He wanted to lose fifteen pounds (surface goal) to have more energy (intrinsic goal) so he could resume playing racquetball with his friends (underlying goal).

Bob started to feel an increase in his energy level, his intrinsic goal, only two weeks after he started exercising — before he had achieved any significant weight loss. Therefore, Bob was motivated to continue so he could see more results. Too many people become frustrated too early if they do not see any progress, often even before they have properly adjusted to their new schedules and changes in habit.

Examples of Extrinsic Goals	Examples of Intrinsic Goals	Examples of Underlying Goals
• losing weight • gaining weight • increasing muscular strength • increasing muscular endurance • increasing cardiovascular capacity • increasing flexibility	• having more energy • achieving a better quality of sleep • feeling less stressed	• increasing self-confidence • feeling good about yourself • cultivating or maintaining friendships • enjoying a better quality of life

Goal Assessment Form

Extrinsic Goals	Intrinsic Goals	Underlying Goals
1	1	1
2	2	2
3	3	3
4	4	4
5	5	5

After you have completed the Goal Assessment Form, take a few minutes to contemplate your underlying goals. These can be the hardest to identify because you must examine your true feelings about yourself and what you need to feel happy and healthy.

Most people are surprised that they have more than the one goal they started with. Now you have a true picture of everything you want to achieve and how succeeding at one goal helps you to reach others.

Breaking Goals Down

*H*ave you ever been faced with an overwhelming task and asked yourself, "How am I ever going to do this?" The more you thought about it, the more uneasy you became. Possibly your anxiety led to the paralysis of inaction: the job just seemed too big to start, much less finish. We can learn a lot about facing daunting challenges from watching children.

Babies who want to explore their surroundings do not just get up one day and start to run around the living room. A baby must first learn to crawl, and then to walk, and then to run — although some parents claim that their child ran first and had to learn how to slow down! If you have ever watched babies when they learn to crawl, you will have noticed that they can come up with unusual ways to reach their goal. Some babies will do the knees-and-elbows crawl while others will scoot across the floor on their rear ends to get to what they want. They then start to pull themselves up on furniture. When they let go and fall, they keep trying again and again until they get to where they want to be. Although there may be the occasional tear, or yelp of frustration, most of the time babies appear to rejoice in the process of mastering new skills one step at a time.

Embrace this attitude when trying to reach your own goals. It will not be easy, but if you stumble, just maintain your sense of humour and keep on trying.

Your smaller goals should be Specific, Measurable, Attainable, Realistic, and Time-oriented. The SMART model is used by health professionals to help their clients stay focused and motivated. Say, for instance, one of your intrinsic goals is to "have more energy." That is a very vague goal. How will you quantify it? If you usually start to feel tired by 7:00 at night, then your goal should be to extend that time to 7:30. If your goal were to extend that time to midnight, it would not be attainable and therefore not realistic. Your goal must also be time-oriented. You need to set a specific deadline by which to attain your goal, otherwise you will be tempted to defer action in favour of other obligations that do carry specific time frames.

Extrinsic goals or surface goals should also be set using the SMART model. If you want to lose twenty pounds, you need to ask yourself whether that is a realistic and attainable goal. If it is, then you need to break down your goal and make it specific. A more specific goal would be to lose one or two pounds per week for a defined period of time. But is this goal truly measurable? Many people get discouraged when the scale doesn't show regular weight loss. But a scale cannot differentiate between fat loss and a corresponding increase in lean muscle. For this reason, you are better off changing the goal into one that can be measured, such as decreasing your percentage of body fat, slimming your waistline, or being able to button your favourite pants.

Underlying or emotional goals must also be realistic. It is not realistic to think that exercise or weight loss will make you a completely happy person. Only you can judge when you feel more confident or have a better quality of life. Tracking the change in your attitude must be a conscious process. That is why it is important to set aside a few minutes at the end of the day to record your feelings in *The Lifetime Journal.** Here you can keep track of all your appointments, and record the type, length, and intensity of your exercise on a daily basis. A checklist of recommended daily servings from all the food groups and a place to record your feelings about the changes you are making in your life are also provided. Every page gives you a daily message of motivation, and each month begins with a new Lifestyle Planning Worksheet and a Lifestyle Planning Checklist so you can identify new barriers and obstacles in the month ahead and put new strategies into action.

When you apply time frames to your goals, remember that there are some events or situations that are out of your control. You may come down with the flu, there could be a crisis at work, or a family member could encounter an emergency and need your help. Be kind to yourself. No matter how well you

---

The Lifetime Journal is the companion book to *Mind Over Matter*. It is designed specifically to help you reach and maintain your exercise and healthy eating habits. To order, please contact Susan Cantwell and Associates by phone at (506) 459-2665, by mail at P.O. Box 591, Station A, Fredericton, NB, Canada E3B 5A6 or by email at scprofit@nbnet.nb.ca.

plan, you cannot anticipate everything that is going to happen. Set your time frames with the understanding that they are flexible. Instead of becoming angry or upset if you do not reach a goal within the time frame you originally set, move it forward.

Case Study *Goals That Matter*

Instant gratification — we all want it, many of us think we *need* it. We are all in a rush to finish something so we can start something new, and begin the cycle again. Such is the case with Yvonne, a twenty-eight-year-old speech pathologist. Between Yvonne's busy social life and work, she does not have any time for exercise and eats at restaurants more often than not. Recently she has noticed that her clothes are again getting a bit tight — she'd already gone up two sizes in the past year and a half. Still, she's not concerned. She knows she can always take the extra weight off when she has the time.

One day, Yvonne receives an invitation to her ten-year high school reunion. She vows to herself that she will lose the extra weight before the reunion, three months away.

A month later, Yvonne steps onto the scale and is horrified to learn that she's thirty-three pounds more than her desired weight. She has only eight weeks until the reunion, so she decides to start jogging again and to go on a diet — no more fattening foods for her.

For the first week, everything seems to be on track. Yvonne starts jogging every night after work. It's not as easy as she remembered and her legs are sore every day. Yvonne also starts to cook more healthy meals at home, rather than eat in restaurants or pick up takeout food. Over the weekend, when Yvonne goes out with her friends, she watches with envy as they eat and drink whatever they want.

On Sunday, Yvonne wakes up and takes a quick shower. Her mind is on one thing and one thing only — today she is going to weigh herself! After six days of exercising and depriving herself of the food she normally eats, she is sure she has lost weight. She steps onto the scale and looks down. One hundred and fifty-six pounds. She has lost three pounds. There must be some mistake. Yvonne steps off the scale and then back on. It reads the same. Yvonne was sure she had lost more weight! At this rate, she will never shed all thirty-three pounds. Yvonne decides to go to the bookstore the next day during her lunch hour to buy a diet book.

On Monday night, after jogging, Yvonne prepares a grocery list of the foods she will need for her diet. She looks at the list again and grimaces. She doesn't like half of the foods in the meal plan. *Oh well*, she thinks, *if I want this weight to come off, I am just going to have to suffer.*

During that week, Yvonne struggles to stick to her new diet. She is always ravenous before it's time to eat and she never feels satisfied after she has finished a meal. She increases her jog from twenty-five to thirty minutes. She is sore and hungry for most of the week, but she does notice that she's not as tired as she usually is at the end of the day.

On the second Sunday after beginning her diet and exercise program, Yvonne steps onto the scale again. One hundred and fifty-four pounds, for a total loss of five pounds. Yvonne curses and stares malevolently at the scale.

That afternoon, Yvonne accepts a lunch invitation from a friend. She orders a meal high in fat and calories. *I will treat myself,* she thinks. *Why should I suffer while my friends eat whatever they please?*

On Monday morning, Yvonne feels guilty about gorging the day before. All day long, she dwells on her lapse until she grows increasingly depressed. That night she has a hard time motivating herself to jog, and she lasts only fifteen minutes. The next day is hectic at work. She has to stay late and decides to pick up her favourite takeout rather than cook. *I will jog twice as long tomorrow,* she thinks, as she sits down in front of the television to eat her supper.

The next day Yvonne restarts her diet, which she refers to as her personal hunger strike. That night she goes to bed hungry. On Friday, Yvonne does not exercise. Instead, she goes out with her friends. She orders a low-fat meal and feels unsatisfied when she finishes. She picks at her friend's nachos while she has a few beers.

On Saturday, Yvonne goes jogging and sticks to her diet; after all, Sunday is weigh-in day.

On the third Sunday of her regimen, the scale display reads 152 pounds. Yvonne has lost only two pounds in a whole week. *This is ridiculous*, she thinks, and goes back to bed.

Yvonne never does lose any more weight. She is unhappier with herself than before she tried to change her lifestyle. She reverts to her previous habits and gains back ten pounds before her reunion. She goes out and buys a new size 16 outfit for the occasion.

A month later Yvonne is asked to attend a retirement party for someone at the hospital where she works. The outfit she wore to her reunion no longer feels right, so she buys another outfit.

Yvonne's first mistake was in setting an unrealistic goal. For Yvonne to reach her goal she would have had to lose just over four pounds per week for eight weeks. A standard safe weight loss is one to two pounds per week. The next problem was that she did not break her goal down into smaller SMART goals. If Yvonne had been realistic about the amount of weight she could lose before her reunion, she would have set her target at sixteen pounds. She would then have broken down that goal into two pounds per week. Her first week's loss of three pounds would have been cause for rejoicing and would have reinforced Yvonne's motivation. She would have felt justified in sticking to her chosen eating plan and not put herself on a highly restrictive diet that she could not expect to sustain.

Yvonne also did not set any intrinsic goals. At the end of her second week, Yvonne noticed that she had more energy at the end of each day, but she did not associate this feeling with any sort of goal, so she disregarded it. Her sole measure of success was the numerals on her scale.

Finally, Yvonne never identified her underlying goal, which was to increase her self-esteem and confidence. Now, whenever Yvonne needs to give her confidence a boost, she just buys a new outfit. She is putting a Band-Aid on her problem while sacrificing her physical and emotional health.

Ten Key Steps to Success

*M*ost people who want to lose weight, to change their body shape, or simply to get fit never look beyond their surface goals. They have not thought about why they want to change or how their appearance shapes how they feel about themselves.

No one is ever 100 percent satisfied with how he or she looks. If you focus entirely on your appearance, you will never achieve complete success. But if you focus on the intrinsic and underlying benefits you will enjoy from exercise and proper eating habits, the changes in your physical appearance will become a side benefit of your efforts.

1 Allow yourself the time to learn how to change certain behaviours.

2 Identify what your surface goal is. This goal is usually the first thing that comes to your mind when you think about why you want to change.

3 Set some intrinsic goals. A great part of how you feel about yourself is based on how you feel on a day-to-day basis.

4 Figure out what your underlying goals are.

5 Evaluate your underlying goals to discover whether they reflect what you truly want. When you know what is truly motivating you to change, you will have a greater chance of success.

6 Understand the relationship between the different types of goals and how attaining one type of goal will lead to attaining the next.

7 Apply reasonable, flexible time frames to your goals.

8 Use the SMART model to set your goals and measure your success.

9 Record your thoughts and feelings each day in the *Lifetime Journal*. Reread what you wrote the day before and look for positive changes in your thoughts and feelings.

10 Be aware that the scale is a limited tool. Do not give it the power to determine your self-worth!

5

Making the Time for Success

$\mathcal{L}$ike everyone these days, you probably lead a hectic life. Sometimes you wonder just how you get it all done. When an unforeseen demand pops up in an already full day, you still manage to fit it in. A forgotten lunch, an unexpected deadline at work, a friend calling to ask for a favour — no problem.

In every family, there seems to be one person who falls into the role of the "fixer." This person assumes the responsibility of making sure that everything gets done and that life runs smoothly for the entire family. If there is a problem, the fixer will sort it out. Fixers automatically pick up the ball when it is dropped and push their needs to the bottom of the list. Often fixers become frustrated because they cannot find time for themselves, but they continue to put their needs last because they fear that if they do not step in, tasks will not be done or will be done improperly.

It can be hard to keep your priorities straight if you are a fixer. But if you are going to successfully achieve your goals, you must learn to reprioritize. Just how important are your goals to you? Isn't it time to take some time for yourself? If your answer is yes, you must rethink your behaviour.

Most of us feel obliged to do *everything* we are asked to. But we need to ask ourselves what the consequences are of not performing a particular task; the consequences of not taking time for our own needs could be far greater than the effects of letting someone else down or not completing the task.

It is often easier to put your needs last than to accept the consequences of disappointing someone else. But this type of behaviour inevitably catches up with you. When you feel that you have no control over your schedule and needs, resentment, frustration, and helplessness ensue. Clinical depression may not be far behind. One way to gain control is to examine your priorities. Is doing the laundry on Monday really more important than exercising? How will doing the laundry tomorrow affect you and your family? Will your son be upset if he does not have his favourite shirt for the next day? Will that scar him for life or will he, after some grumbling, just put on another shirt?

If reaching your health goals is important to you, then you must give exercise and eating properly a high priority in your life. One of the best ways to incorporate exercise into your schedule is to look for ways to be more active as part of your day-to-day routine. If your workplace is close enough, walk or bike to work instead of driving. Take the stairs instead of the elevator. If one of your children is involved in a sport, volunteer to coach or referee instead of watching from the sidelines. If you use a riding lawnmower, get out your old push mower. There are countless ways to fit fitness into your life, even in our convenience-laden world.

Another way to make exercise and eating properly a priority is to schedule appointments with *yourself* right in your day planner. If someone asks you to do something on Friday at noon and there is already a written appointment in that time slot, you can truthfully say that you have a prior commitment. You are not being selfish; you are simply recognizing the need to take care of yourself, along with the others you look after.

Exercising and taking care of yourself are among the most unselfish actions you can take because your health directly affects the people you love. If you continue to lead an unhealthy life, how will it affect your family if you become seriously ill?

Sometimes it takes a life-or-death event to get us to understand that eating properly and exercising must be given top priority. The illness of a friend or family member brings what we think is important in our lives into perspective. Have you ever heard of a dying person who expressed regret that he did not spend enough time at the office?

How you choose to spend your time is key to achieving your goals. Every time you agree to a new activity, that activity will subtract from your personal time. There is a price to be paid for each new commitment you make. The cost is your time. When you take on too much, your efforts are scattered or diluted. When you are trying to change behaviours, having a lot on your plate makes it harder to meet your goals. In the cycle of success, allocating the time to achieve consistency is one of the stepping stones to results. The way you manage your time will either help you reach your goals or hinder your efforts.

Just Say No

It's short and simple but "no" can be one of the hardest words to say. Can you count the number of times over the last year that you did something that you did not want to do or agreed to do something you regretted later? If you did manage to say no, did you follow up the refusal with a long explanation and feel uncomfortable? Learning to say no — and not feeling guilty about it — is a vital survival skill.

The first step to learning to say no is to practise saying it. Say no in the shower, repeat it on your walk or drive to work, look in the mirror and say it to yourself. The next step is to understand what your schedule and commitments are on a day-to-day and week-to-week basis. If you are not sure that you have the time to respond to someone's request, do not allow yourself to feel pressured into saying yes. If you need to look over your schedule, tell the person that you will get back to him or her as soon as possible.

Sometimes when we say yes, what we thought was a one-hour commitment turns into a two- or three-hour commitment. Make sure you understand what is being asked of you. Ask questions like, "How much of my time will this require?" or "What will be expected of me?" If you do want to help, but cannot do the entire task, place conditions on your agreement: "I cannot sit on the committee for the book drive, but I can man the table for two hours on the day of the book sale."

If you determine that you do not have the time, use the word "no" when you are declining; don't fudge by saying "I don't think so." If you use terms like "I don't think so," you leave the door open for further persuasion and, with that, further pressure. Be firm when you refuse. Too often when we say no, we do so while smiling or nodding our heads yes. Make sure your non-verbal gestures are consistent with your spoken answer.

When you do decide to say no, do not feel tempted to go into a long, drawn-out explanation of why you are refusing the request. Your explanation just offers opportunities for the asker to sort out your schedule for you. Be as brief as possible; use sentences like, "No, I can't. My schedule is full."

People can be very persuasive when they are in a bind because of their own poor planning and time-management skills. Do not let them make their problems your problems. If you have to say no, but really would like to help, try to redirect the request to someone who might be able to lend a hand: "No, I can't. My schedule is full. Why don't you check with Emily or Sam, and see what their schedules are like?"

Never let anyone try to make you feel guilty about saying no. People will tell you they have asked everyone else and you are their last hope. This is just a blatant attempt to make you take ownership of their problem. When people cannot resolve a situation by finding someone to help them, they must adjust their own schedules to get the task done. We have all had to do this at one time or another; the person who is pressuring you may need to be encouraged to consider this option.

Try to be realistic about the consequences of taking on another task that interferes with your priorities. Do not feel guilty about refusing if you did not create the problem or task in the first place. ***You are not responsible for solving other people's problems or shortcomings***.

From childhood, we learn that "no" is a negative barrier to the things we want, but denying requests or demands for your time is a step towards making "no" a positive factor in your own life. When you say no, you are actually saying, "*Yes*, I am worth the time it will take to lead a healthier and happier life."

Identifying Time Thieves

One universal complaint about time is that there never seems to be enough of it. Everyone struggles with the restrictions of time. You have heard the expressions "a race against the clock" and "working on a deadline." We think of time as an enemy in our lives, limiting and controlling what we are able to accomplish. Yet time is our most valuable non-renewable resource. Once we have wasted time, we cannot go out and buy some more. We can replace clothes, cars, furniture, and even spouses, but not time.

How you spend your time is how you choose to live your life. What does your life say about the way you manage your time? Time is not the enemy, but something to be treasured. If time is truly valuable, shouldn't you use it to do things that make yourself and the people you love happier and healthier?

Most of us use our time-management skills only to fulfil our essential responsibilities. We fail to recognize the time thieves in our day-to-day lives. It is amazing how much extra time we can free up in our schedules by identifying and redirecting or eliminating our personal time thieves. These time thieves can be co-workers, friends, or even relatives. They can also be people you do not even know. These people invade your life without notice and say, "Listen to me right now." Most of us do.

For example, you are just about to leave your house for an appointment. You have your coat on, your car keys in one hand, and your other hand is on the doorknob when the telephone rings. You immediately stop, turn around, and rush back to answer the telephone. The caller is a friend who wants to ask you a question. "I am just on my way out the door," you say.

"I just have a question. It won't take a minute," your friend replies.

Does it ever really take "just a minute"? Are you picturing someone in your mind right now — someone who calls and then continues the conversation even when you make repeated attempts to get off the telephone?

Another of your time thieves could be a co-worker who comes into your office for legitimate reasons but lingers to chat. Another co-worker may interrupt you because she is always in the midst of a crisis due to poor planning. Relatives can also be time thieves if they make unfair or unreasonable demands on your time when there are other people available to help them. We let time thieves interfere with our priorities and schedules because we do not want to disappoint or offend them. But if you constantly allow someone to take up your time, they will come to believe that you accept or even welcome their intrusions. Some desperate and creative people have come up with ingenious strategies to deal with chatty phone friends, such as getting a spouse to call them from across the room — or even ringing their own doorbells! The problem with these subterfuges is that they do not change the behaviour of the person who repeatedly squanders your time.

By now, you will have identified your time thieves. Here are some helpful tips to deal with them and give you the time you need to accomplish what is important to you.

The Chatty Friend

- Ignore the telephone — it is a tool, and you can choose to answer it or not. You don't have to answer just because it rings!
- Get call display. You will be able to see if the telephone call is a priority or if it can wait.
- Use voice mail to screen your calls.
- Place a time restriction on the call at the beginning of it. "I can only talk for five minutes." After five minutes, politely but firmly end the call.
- Don't waffle by saying "I guess I should get off the telephone," or "I should go now." Use phrases like "I am going to go now. Thank you for calling. Good-bye."

The Demanding Friend or Relative

- Ask yourself why you always say yes to this particular person. Once you have a better understanding of why you have allowed this pattern of behaviour to persist, you will be better equipped to change it.
- Acknowledge the other person's disappointment at your refusal with phrases like "I know this will be disappointing, but I can't help you right now."
- Don't apologize. You have nothing to be sorry for.

- Redirect the relative to another family member or friend who might be able to help.
- If you have no alternative, say that you will help this one time, but stress that you will not be available on a regular basis.

The Co-worker in Crisis

- Establish whether there really is a crisis. Some people live in a state of crisis or exaggerate their problems.
- If there is no crisis, schedule a meeting at a more convenient time.
- Whenever possible, refer your colleague to someone else in the company who can help them.
- Give the co-worker a time limit when he or she comes to your office. "I can give you five minutes; I've got to get back to this file."
- Stand up — it will signal that you are finished listening. If necessary, walk the time thief to the door.

These simple yet effective time-management tips can provide you with the extra time you need to get your work done and free you up to meet your personal priorities.

Learning How to Share the Load

When it comes to running a household, there are a series of tasks that are never finished because they must be done over and over again. Vacuuming the floor, cleaning the bathrooms, doing the laundry, buying groceries, cooking, making lunches, taking out the garbage, and mowing the lawn are all chores that need to be done on a day-to-day or week-to-week basis. At the beginning of a relationship, people fall into a routine for getting these tasks done. Usually, if one person is staying at home, he or she assumes the majority of the domestic tasks. If both partners work, the tasks should be evenly divided. But quite often, during the course of a relationship, the division becomes unbalanced, with one person doing more than the other.

This imbalance evolves for a number of reasons. One person may experience a temporary increase in workload, leading the other to take over some of their tasks. When a woman goes on maternity leave she may assume almost all of the household tasks *and* take care of the new baby. When she returns to work outside the home, she may continue to do most household jobs. If either partner is laid off or has a sabbatical, he or she may assume a larger role at home, which persists even after the return to work. This imbalance is usually not a deliberate effort to avoid doing a fair share, but rather is the result of a lack of communication between partners.

If chores are split unevenly in your household, you need to work to re-establish balance. What you do inside the household is usually a reflection of how your parents divided up household tasks. It is important to understand your partner's background before you try to balance the workload.

The first step to creating more balance is to talk with your partner in a non-confrontational manner. Phrases like "I am doing all the work" or "You are not doing enough" create antagonism. Your partner will become defensive and an argument will usually ensue. The best way to gain cooperation is to write up a list of all the household duties, inside and out, and start by saying, "I need your help. I am having a hard time getting everything done." Take out your list. Ask your partner what he or she expects of you, and then tell your partner what you need from him or her. Go over the list and ask which tasks your partner prefers doing. Do the same yourself, then come to an agreement about how to divide the chores neither of you cares for. Once you have divided the tasks fairly, thank your partner and post the list where you will both see it.

The same process can be used with your children. Many parents fall into the trap of performing household tasks for their children when they are little, and continue to perform them even when the children are old enough to assume their own responsibilities. Sit down with your children and show them the entire list of the tasks you and your partner perform and request their help. Have the children pick which tasks they will be responsible for. This is a valuable tool for teaching your children about working together as a family and sharing responsibility.

In the beginning, your partner or your children might need a reminder to do these new tasks. Politely but firmly remind them of the task, but do not perform the task for them. If you do, you will teach them that if they fail to do a task you will do it for them.

If you follow through with this process, the result will be a fairer distribution of the household duties, which will help you create more balance in your life.

Case Study *Taking Responsibility — for Everyone Else*

"It's an emergency," Charlotte pleads. "I have to take Mark to hockey practice and the baby's sick." Mary sighs as she sits back in her office chair and stares at the files in front of her. With her sister, it's always an emergency. Mary glances at her watch. She has five minutes before she has to get to a meeting and she still has to sort through her files.

"What about Tom?" Mary asks about Charlotte's husband.

"He has to work late. He won't be home in time and I can't take Julie to a cold arena when she is sick. Could you come over right after work? I'll only be an hour and a half. Tom might even get home sooner than that."

Mary had planned to exercise right after work. "Well, I'm really busy —" Mary says evasively.

"Can you do it?" Charlotte asks, in a rush. Mary looks at her watch again. She's going to be late for her meeting.

"All right. I'll be there after work."

"Thanks a lot. I'll see you then." Mary hangs up the telephone, quickly sifts through her files, and races off to her meeting.

After the meeting, Mary comes back to her office. She has not gotten half the work done that she wanted to that morning. She decides to work through lunch to get back on track, so she won't have to take work home. She gets a lot accomplished and has only three more things to get done by the end of the day. She is just starting to catch her breath when there is a knock on her door.

"Hi. Do you have a minute?" Jim asks, coming in and sitting down across the desk from her. "Could you look over these figures for me? This purchasing report is due at the end of the week and something doesn't make sense." Jim places a report on Mary's desk and opens it. Though Mary does not work in Jim's department, she is always able to spot problems quickly. The two co-workers spend half an hour going over the report before Mary discovers the source of the problem. She gives Jim the proper figures.

"Thanks. I knew you would find it. I don't know why I didn't see the problem," Jim sits back, relaxed. "You look swamped," Jim says belatedly, as he eyes the top on Mary's desk.

"Aren't I always?" Mary replies, glancing furtively at her watch. She has just lost the hour she made up by working through lunch and now she's hungry.

"Working on anything interesting?"

"No. Just the usual stuff," Mary says, trying to keep the conversation short.

"Did you hear that Allan is leaving?" Jim offers, proceeding to tell Mary at length about Allen's transfer. By the time Jim finally leaves, Mary has lost another half-hour. There is no way she can get everything done by 5:00. She's going to have to take work home. Mary hates days like this, when it seems she just can't get anything done. *So much for exercising,* she thinks.

Mary leaves work at 5:00 and drives to her sister's house to babysit. She heats up some leftover macaroni-and-cheese casserole that Charlotte had prepared for supper. It's not what she would have preferred to eat since it is loaded with fat.

Tom does not get home before her sister gets back; by the time Mary leaves it is 7:30. It takes her half an hour to drive home. By the time she sits down to finish the work she brought home, it is after 9:00. She has not exercised as she had planned or eaten properly. Mary passes off her lapses as "having a bad day." She will have a lot more bad days until she changes the way she manages her time.

Do you see where Mary let other people take up the time she had allotted to getting her own work done so she could eat properly and exercise? Mary wanted to help her sister but she could have helped her in a different way.

She could have made it clear from the beginning of the conversation that she had something else scheduled and offered helpful suggestions to her sister, such as getting another parent to give her son a lift to hockey practice. Had her sister tried a babysitter? Could her son miss one practice?

In the case of her co-worker, Jim, Mary could have made it clear that she had only five minutes to devote to his problem. She could have redirected him to someone else in his own department or scheduled a meeting with him for sometime later in the week.

Mary solved everyone else's problems and, in the course of doing so, created stress for herself. If she does not start to change the way she deals with her time thieves, she will never have the time to make her desired lifestyle changes. Her sister and her co-workers will never attempt to solve their own problems because they know that they can always fall back on Mary.

If you do want to help someone, by all means do so. But if a person makes repeated demands on your time and interferes with the way you want to lead your life, it is time for you to firmly and politely say no.

Ten Key Steps to Success

Most of us have time in our schedules to exercise and eat properly if we manage our time correctly. Are you willing to make changes in your life to get the time? Change can be difficult, especially for people who are used to pleasing others and putting their own needs last. When you are constantly called on to fix other people's problems, you help neither yourself nor them in the long run. They will never have to face the consequences of their poor planning, and you will never be able to reach your goals. You will be amazed at how easy it is to manage your time more effectively once you start choosing who gets to use it.

Another benefit to effective time management is increased self-esteem. Being able to express your wishes and avoiding situations that cause you stress will enhance your well-being.

1   Establish your priorities and make appointments with yourself in your day planner.

2   Highlight tasks or appointments in your day planner that must be completed that day, *including* eating properly and exercising.

3   Look for ways to incorporate more exercise into your daily routine. Every little bit counts.

4   Practice saying the word "no."

5   Be firm and do not apologize for problems that are not your own.

6   Don't feel pressured into saying yes if you are not sure how a task will affect the rest of your schedule.

7   Identify your own personal time thieves and evaluate why you say yes to their repeated demands for your time.

8   Write a list of everything that needs to be done inside and outside the home. Have a family meeting to discuss the household duties and allow others to choose what tasks they want to do each week.

9   Post the list and review it regularly.

10   Do not revert to completing other people's tasks unless there is a *specific* reason to do so and they are made aware of your help.

6

Knowledge Is Power

*W*hen you think about starting something new, you may have some preconceptions about the new activity. If you have had a negative experience with a particular activity, your feelings about trying it again will be negative. If in university you had a tedious psychology professor who spoke in a monotone, you probably perceive psychology as boring. The same can be said for previous attempts to exercise or eat properly. If you felt discomfort while exercising, constant hunger while trying to change your eating habits, or if you did not get the results you wanted, you probably think that exercising and eating properly are impossible feats. But if you understand the process your body will go through and the feelings you will experience, you will be better prepared to deal with them.

Shelley started to walk three times a week around her neighbourhood. She had been thinking about improving her fitness since her thirty-fifth birthday four years ago, and was determined to stick with her decision to lose the ten extra pounds she had been carrying for the last six years. Shelley was now ready to start and felt optimistic about her decision. On Mondays, Wednesdays, and Fridays, she set aside an hour to walk. She dug out her old track suit and running shoes and placed them at the bottom of her bed the night before her first walk.

She set off on Monday morning. She had decided to start slowly and walk only until she was slightly tired, because she did not want to overdo it. She decided to walk down her street, down a hill to another street, and then loop back up the hill to reach her street again. She figured this walk would probably take her fifteen to twenty minutes. Shelley completed her walk without much difficulty and felt refreshed.

"That wasn't too bad," she reflected, as she made herself some breakfast. "This is going to be easier than I thought. I'll go out again tomorrow, instead of waiting till Wednesday."

The next day, when Shelley got out of bed she felt pain in her shins. Every time she took a step, it hurt. There was no way Shelley was going to be able to walk today. She decided to rest and walk again on Wednesday, as she had originally planned.

On Wednesday, Shelley's shins were still bothering her but not as much. She started her walk off slowly and followed the same route that she had on Monday. After she finished walking her legs felt better — until she got up the next day. Again, Shelley had pain in her shins and felt as though she could hardly walk. She decided to make an appointment with her doctor to find out what was wrong.

Her doctor told her to ice her shins and not to resume walking until the pain disappeared. It took two days for her legs to feel better and she took an additional day off just to be safe. Shelley started walking again only to have the same thing happen. By now Shelley was growing discouraged. She started the process of resting and icing her legs again. She did not go out walking for another week, and when she did, the same cycle of pain recurred. Shelley abandoned her resolve for the time being.

Six months later, Shelley's friend Ruth asked her to walk with her three times a week. Shelley declined and told Ruth about her experiences with the pain in her lower legs when she had tried walking in the past. Ruth suggested that if she tried it once and the pain recurred, then she could stop. Shelley agreed but was not hopeful that this time would be any different. That afternoon Shelley and Ruth went out and bought new walking shoes.

The next morning Ruth chose their route and, mindful of Shelley's previous pain, suggested they take it slowly. They walked for about twenty minutes.

The next day Shelley got out of bed expecting the worst. She gingerly put her feet on the floor and stood up. No pain. She took a few steps and still felt no pain. Shelley walked with her friend three to four times a week and they gradually increased their time to forty-five minutes.

Shelley did not understand why her legs were not bothering her, but the reason was simple. The route her friend had chosen did not involve walking up a hill. When Shelley walked by herself, she walked up a steep hill at the end of her walk. Every time Shelley flexed her foot to take a step up the hill, she had to use the muscles in the front part of her lower legs. The hill was at the end of her walk when these muscles were already tiring. Shelley had also been wearing her old running shoes, which gave her no support or cushion from the impact of walking.

If Ruth had not talked her into walking, it might have been years before she tried any form of exercise again. If she had thought to buy new shoes before starting, and had delayed incorporating hills into her walking until she had become more conditioned, she probably would have had a better experience the first time around.

Today Shelley walks for more than an hour each day. She has lost the ten pounds that she wanted to, but says she gets something even more valuable from her walking. "I get a feeling of being totally healthy while I walk. All the jumble of the day's activities seems to fall away and everything shifts into perspective. I feel better about myself and I would not give up walking for anything. I walk off any frustrations and stress. I truly think I am a more balanced person because of walking."

If you intend to start exercising and eating properly, it is essential that you educate yourself about the type of exercise that you have chosen and about preparing and eating things that are healthier for you. The more you know, the more positive an experience you will have with the lifestyle changes you have chosen.

In the rest of this chapter we will look at some of the most common misconceptions about exercise, eating, and weight loss, and give you the facts. Remember: anyone who is going to change exercise and/or eating habits should consult a physician before beginning.

Exercise Basics

$\mathcal{T}$o receive the most health benefit from exercise, you need to understand what types of exercise you should do, and what results they will give you. There are five different physical components of fitness that make up a well-balanced fitness program.

The Warm-Up

Warming up your entire body with cardiovascular exercises and stretching minimizes your risk of injury. A warm-up should begin by gradually increasing your heart rate before you begin the actual workout you have planned. For example, if you plan to go for a run for twenty minutes, you should begin by walking briskly for five to ten minutes. Because your muscles are more easily stretched when they are warm, always stretch after warming up your muscles. You should stretch your calf muscles, hamstrings, quadriceps, and Achilles tendons before actually running. Hold each stretch for fifteen to thirty seconds. Even if your chosen activity is a low-key recreational sport like golf, you should still warm up before playing. You will not only reduce your risk of injury but will also be able to swing the golf club through a greater range of motion to improve your shot. Stretches for muscles that will be used to perform a specific activity are also important.

Cardiovascular Conditioning

Cardiovascular endurance, sometimes referred to as cardiorespiratory endurance, is the ability of the heart and lungs to deliver oxygen to the working muscles for a sustained period. Cardiovascular conditioning is a crucial component in a fitness program because weakened heart muscles put you at an increased risk for heart disease, high blood pressure, diabetes, and many other preventable diseases. Performing some sort of cardiovascular conditioning has many benefits, including better overall health, weight control, increase or maintenance of bone density, reducing stress levels, and heightened energy.

When people think of cardiovascular activities, they usually think of walking or running, but there are many options to choose from. When you choose an activity, make sure that it is something you will enjoy and be willing to do on a consistent basis. If you grow bored with your activity, switch to a new one. Walking, jogging, running, biking, skating, tennis, swimming, dancing, hiking, and group exercise classes are all options. Group exercise classes now offer more diversified and varied programming to include cycling, treadmill walking, and rowing. You can also purchase exercise equipment for your home if you like the convenience and privacy of exercising alone. Whatever activity you choose, make sure that you start out slowly and gradually increase your intensity and duration.

Exercise initially two to three times a week. As you get stronger and feel an increase in your energy, you should try to incorporate at least twenty to thirty minutes of cardiovascular activity into each day (not including your warm-up or cool-down period), four to seven days a week.

Muscular Endurance and Strength

Muscular endurance is the ability of a muscle or muscle group to exert repeated force or to hold a static muscle contraction over a period of time. An example of good muscular endurance is being able to carry your grocery bags across a large parking lot and load them into the car without having your arms tire.

Muscular strength is the maximum force that a muscle can produce against resistance in a single effort. An example of muscular strength is the ability to lift a heavy box. Muscular strength and endurance enable you to perform everyday activities without strain for longer periods before tiring. To maintain a good balance among your upper body, trunk, and lower body, make sure to perform exercises for all your muscle groups. Running or walking builds up muscular strength and endurance only in your lower body, so you should supplement your running/walking program with some upper body and trunk exercises. Also, remember to exercise muscle groups at both the front and the back of your body evenly.

The benefits of muscular strength and endurance are decreased risk of osteoporosis, better posture, improved shapeliness and toning, and an increased sense of well-being.

Some activities that increase muscular strength and endurance are weight-lifting, heavy yard work, yoga, tai chi, push-ups and curls-ups, backpacking, and rock climbing. If you have been inactive for a while, any exercise will help increase the strength and endurance in the muscles you are using.

Try to incorporate some sort of muscular endurance and strength exercises into your day at least twice a week. As you get stronger, you can increase this to three or four times a week. You should never train the same muscle group two days in a row. Remember always to perform exercises with the proper form and technique and to breathe regularly while performing an exercise — never hold your breath. If you are unsure how to perform an exercise, schedule a session with a personal fitness trainer or consult a book. If you feel you need the help of a fitness professional on an ongoing basis, call your local fitness facility to see if there is a program or class you might want to try.

Cool-down

The cool-down is an important part of any exercise program. The purpose of a cool-down is to gradually reduce your heart rate, which has been increased during exercise. A cool-down should immediately follow any form of cardio-vascular exercise such as brisk walking, biking, swimming, or running. A cool-down will help prevent the pooling of blood in the veins. If you stop suddenly you could experience lightheadedness and may even faint. Cooling down also helps reduce muscle soreness after exercise. If you have decided to walk briskly for ten to twenty minutes, then you should slow your pace to a saunter for at least five minutes before you stop. The longer or more intensely you exercise, the longer the cool-down should be. If you run for thirty minutes, you should allow for a five- to ten-minute cool-down.

Flexibility

Flexibility is the range of motion that is possible around any joint. People who have poor flexibility are more prone to injury due to stiff or tight muscles. Because it occurs at the end of a workout when fatigue or time pressures kick in, stretching after a workout is the most overlooked component of a well-balanced fitness program. The benefits of stretching far outweigh the time it takes: an increase in efficiency in your day-to-day activities, decreased risk of injury, increased blood supply to the joints, increased body awareness and lowered stress levels.

A stretching routine should involve stretches for all your muscle groups. If you are short on time you can stretch only the muscles that you have used. You can gain flexibility from yoga, tai chi, or some types of dance classes.

Keep in mind the following tips:

- Hold each stretch for sixty to ninety seconds.
- Stretching should never be painful. If you feel pain or your muscle starts to shake, you are over-stretching.
- Never bounce while stretching. This can cause injury.
- Always breathe regularly while stretching. Do not hold your breath.

After reading this, you might conclude that a well-balanced fitness program will take up a lot of your time. But each exercise session should take you no more than forty-five minutes to an hour to complete, and as you become more familiar with the routine you will move through it more quickly and confidently. Another added benefit to exercising regularly is that the more physically fit you become, the less time you will have to spend exercising. You will be able to exercise at a higher intensity and still derive the same benefits.

Common Exercise Misconceptions

People have a lot of misconceptions about how exercise should feel, how they should feel about exercise, and what kind of results they should get for their efforts. These misconceptions can cause even the most dedicated people to feel that they are wasting their time and energy for little or no return.

1. *Everyone I know who exercises says that they enjoy it. I have just started exercising and I do not enjoy it. What's wrong with me?*
Nothing is wrong with you. Many people do not enjoy exercise when they first start a program. Feeling unsure and tired can add to your perception that

you do not like to exercise. People who have been exercising for a period of time start to enjoy it because they feel an increase in their energy levels and they have got into a comfortable routine. If you stick with your chosen exercise routine for at least a month, you will start to see and feel the benefits of what you are doing. If, after a month, you still do not enjoy exercising, switch to a different activity. Maybe it is not exercise that you do not like but rather the activity you have chosen. If after changing your activity you find you still do not enjoy exercising, think about exercise as a necessary activity in your life such as brushing your teeth. Few people think about whether they enjoy brushing their teeth; they simply know that it is the only way to prevent tooth decay. It is curious that we think we have a choice about whether or not to exercise.

2. *I cannot get motivated to exercise. Am I just lazy?*
Most people have to push themselves to start and, in the following months, to stick with an exercise program. Many create mental barriers, focusing on how busy they are or how cold it is outside. Once you are exercising regularly, you will realize that it is not as difficult as you thought. The feelings of well-being, relaxation, and accomplishment that arise from exercising are what keep most people coming back for more. Try to focus on how good you will feel when you finish and not on the exercise itself.

3. *I do abdominal curls every day to flatten my stomach, but I cannot see any results. What am I doing wrong?*
Many people believe that they can target a specific area of their bodies and get results just from performing muscular endurance exercises such as ab curls. If this were true, people who talked a lot would all have thin faces! While ab curls will help you lose inches off your stomach, you will not see the results of your efforts until you reduce your overall body fat. Unless you combine abdominal exercises with cardiovascular conditioning activities such as walking, exercise classes, or biking, you will not achieve the results you seek.

4. *I am a woman and I have been hearing a lot about the benefits of resistance training over the last couple of years. Can I do weight training without ending up with big, bulky muscles?*

Resistance training is a great way to tone and firm your body and, when combined with cardiovascular conditioning, it will help you maintain or lose weight. The fear that women will develop big, bulky muscles from weight training is unwarranted. If you want to strengthen, firm, and tone your muscles you should perform ten to twelve repetitions of an exercise for each muscle group and work your way up to three sets of each exercise. Bulking up, as practised by bodybuilders, is the result of a much more demanding weight-training regimen and of dietary changes and supplements that are not recommended for the ordinary exerciser.

5. *I am so sore the day after I work out that I have a hard time moving without pain. I have heard that if you do not feel the muscles you have worked the next day, you are not doing enough. Is this true?*

Absolutely not! This myth probably got started in the bodybuilding gyms of the 1980s. Bodybuilders need to lift heavy weights with few repetitions in order to increase the size of a particular muscle. The muscle needs to be worked to exhaustion, an unpleasant feeling that bodybuilders refer to as "feeling the burn." The bodybuilders' "no pain, no gain" philosophy filtered into the general population, where it has had dangerous consequences. Responsible group exercise leaders try to balance safety with what the participants in their classes perceive to be a "good" workout. But instructors who push and cajole their participants to "feel the burn" are often rewarded with larger attendance figures than those who provide a safer, less intense workout, and the myth of "no pain, no gain" is further perpetuated.

Exercise should *never* be painful. Pain is your body's way of warning you to stop. While a certain amount of delayed muscle soreness is to be expected when you start or change an exercise program, this discomfort should not interfere with your daily tasks. If you are experiencing pain, you may be trying to exceed your current fitness level, performing an exercise with poor technique, or not stretching after exercising. You might also have an underlying condition, such as a joint or muscular problem, that is aggravated by certain types of exercise. Consult a qualified health/fitness professional and/or your physician if you are experiencing chronic exercise-related pain.

Common Diet Dilemmas

𝒲hy is it so difficult to stick to a diet? Every time a new diet comes out, people rush to get on it because they believe that the reason they have failed in the past has to do with the diet they were on. They are partly right, but there is no reason to assume that this new diet will help them achieve the results they want. If a diet is highly restrictive it will be harder to follow and maintain. No one can live like a saint for the rest of his or her life. When you are looking for a diet to help you lose weight, it should be one that you feel comfortable with eating forever, not just until you lose weight. A major problem with most diets is that you see results almost immediately because they are so restrictive. After you reach your goal, you start to eat normally again and gain all your weight back. If we have learned anything from the last ten years, it is that *diets do not work* for long-term weight management.

Gradually cutting down on foods with high fat content and increasing your intake of healthy foods like fruits and vegetables is the only realistic, effective way to diet. The key word is *gradually*. The more drastic the changes you make in your eating habits, the more difficult you will find it to stick with them permanently. You can still have the foods you enjoy. If you usually eat three cookies a day, cut one out until you are satisfied with just two, then move gradually toward one a day, one every other day, and so on.

Many people who change to a low-fat diet still have trouble losing weight. The problem lies not with what they are eating but rather with how much they are eating. What we require and what we consume are not the same. The formula for weight loss is simple. If you eat more calories than you expend, you are going to gain weight. If your calorie intake is the same as the calories you expend, you will maintain your weight, and if your calorie intake is less than the calories you expend, you will lose weight. It is as simple as that.

As children, we are taught to eat everything on our plates and this early message is carried into adulthood. Many adults eat oversized portions of just about everything. Do you ever wonder why your child has a hard time finishing a meal in a restaurant? Most family restaurants want you to feel that you are getting good value for your money so they give you oversized portions. What many people believe are correct portions of food are actually oversized by 10 to 25 percent. The combined perceptions that oversized portions are normal and that we must finish everything on our plates make it difficult for people to lose weight.

Here are ten helpful hints for eating properly:

1. Identify the foods you eat that are high in fat and plan to gradually decrease the amount of one of these foods each month.
2. Drink six to eight eight-ounce glasses of water a day.
3. Look at the size of your dinner plates. If they are large, replace them with smaller plates filled with smaller portions. You will feel as if you are eating the same amount of food even though there is less on your plate.
4. Start your meal off with soup, which will help fill you up so you will not feel the urge to overeat.
5. Chew your food slowly and put down your fork and knife while chewing.
6. Stop eating when you feel slightly full, even if there is still food on your plate.
7. If you want to have a snack, ask yourself if you are really hungry. Many people eat out of boredom or habit.
8. Keep a daily food journal for at least a week. Write down everything that you eat and drink, the time of day, and what you were doing. This will help you to see exactly what you are eating, what times of day you tend to eat, and what activities you associate with eating, so you can cut back on those activities or schedule exercise during that time.
9. Stop and think about whether you are really hungry if someone offers you food. Don't automatically accept the proffered goodies just to be polite.
10. Never go on a diet that requires you to consume less than 1,200 calories a day for a woman or 1,800 calories a day for a man.

If you feel you need the structure of a mass-market diet, avoid those that eliminate any of the food groups. That kind of diet might rob you of important nutrients that your body needs. Never skip breakfast. If you don't eat breakfast, it may be harder for you to lose weight. Your body and your metabolism need a kick-start in the morning after eight to twelve hours of no food.

Case Study *What You Don't Know <u>Can</u> Hurt You*

At age forty-nine, James thought he was ready for a change. His waist size had gotten larger over the years, along with his paycheque! James was a successful lawyer who worked a twelve-hour day, leaving time for little else. He had taken his share of vacations over the years with his wife and two children, now teenagers. He always came back more relaxed than when he had left, but could not seem to regain the same energy level he felt when he was younger.

I must be getting old, James thought as he sat down behind the desk in his office to read some briefs. He could not concentrate; he was tired. *Maybe I am coming down with something*. He scanned his appointments for the day. Nothing was crucial.

James's wife, Jennifer, was surprised to see him in the middle of the day. "What are you doing home?" she asked.

"I'm just so tired," James said, looking around the kitchen.

"Do you feel sick?" Jennifer felt his forehead.

"No, just tired."

"Well, I hate to tell you this, James, but you are always tired." Jennifer sat down across from him. "I think it's time you started to think about getting some exercise," she urged for the thousandth time.

Here we go again, thought James. As Jennifer talked, James's mind started to drift. *Maybe she's right, maybe I should start to exercise*. "You're right," he said. "Tomorrow I'll join that fitness club near the office."

The next day James did join the fitness club. He made an appointment to meet with a fitness consultant the following week. But on the day of his appointment he had to cancel because he was backed up at work. Not to be deterred from starting to exercise, James decided to go to the club anyway.

James decided that the stationary bike would be his best bet. He went in and biked for ten minutes before he felt he should stop. Pleased that he had started, he did not set up another appointment to design a personalized program with the fitness consultant.

After about a month, James started to feel an increase in his energy level and had lost about three pounds. Jennifer was pleased with the effort he was making; the program seemed to be going well. James was a bit sore after each one of his workouts but thought that was because he was out of shape. The worst pain was in his back, which ached constantly. It was annoying, but James was sure the pain would go away once he got in better shape.

One night, Jennifer remembered that the fitness club had called about two weeks before to reschedule James's original appointment. James told her he didn't think he needed to speak to the consultant: he knew what he was doing.

After three months, James had lost twelve pounds. His back was still bothering him but he felt pleased with his accomplishment. If his back would only stop hurting so much, he could increase his exercise level, try to lose more weight, and expect to feel even better.

One day, during the third month of his new routine, James was in his office working and he dropped his pen. Bending over to pick it up, he felt a sharp pain in his lower back and was unable to straighten up.

James had to be helped from his office. He was driven immediately to his doctor's office, where he was told he had strained his lower back. He was prescribed muscle relaxants and told to rest for at least four days.

It took James six days to be able to walk properly, and even then he still felt pain. During physiotherapy he was told he had tight hamstrings and that because he did not stretch before and after his workouts, these tight muscles had contributed to his lower back problems.

It took James four months to start exercising at his fitness facility again. By then he had gained back all of the weight he had lost. This time he kept his appointment with the fitness consultant and was given a well-balanced fitness program. He learned why it was important to stretch before and after every workout and how to stretch properly. James realized that if he had kept his initial appointment, or had some knowledge about the essential components of a fitness program, he would not have injured himself nor regained his lost weight. Now he had to start all over again.

James did eventually lose the weight he wanted to and feels even better than when he was thirty-five. Nevertheless, he says, he nearly did not resume his exercise program.

"When I first hurt my back, I thought it was because I was at the age when my body was starting to give out. After I talked to the physiotherapist, I realized that years of inactivity had weakened my muscles and that not stretching after my workouts was dangerous. If I had known how important stretching was, I certainly would have done it."

Ten Key Steps to Success

The more you know about the way your body works and responds to exercise and eating properly, the better chance you have of successfully and permanently changing your life. Take the time to read about exercise and healthy eating practices before you begin a change in your lifestyle. It is not enough to know what you have to do; you need to understand why it should be done.

1 Think of your past experiences as practice for your present lifestyle changes.

2 Reflect on your previous experience with trying to eat a healthy diet and exercise consistently. Try to determine what inhibited you.

3 Consult your physician before beginning an exercise program or making a change in your eating habits.

4 Pick an activity that you enjoy. If you become bored with your chosen fitness program, change the program or activity to something new.

5   Take the time to incorporate a warm-up before you perform any physical activity, and a cool-down, including stretching, after you finish.

6   Purchase appropriate attire and footwear before beginning any fitness program. You might not notice how much cushioning and support your current running shoes have lost until you put on a new pair.

7   Make changes in your diet gradually. Do not deprive yourself of something you enjoy, just eat less of it.

8   Understand that it is normal not to feel motivated to exercise or eat properly every day. If you dwell on your lack of motivation, the task will seem more difficult than it actually is. Just do it without asking yourself if you feel like it.

9   Expect some muscular soreness when you begin an exercise program or new activity, but do not ignore pain. Exercise should *never* be painful.

10 Read everything you can on healthy living. Not only will you gain a better understanding of what you are doing but you will also find that your new knowledge will motivate you to continue with your chosen lifestyle changes.

7

Being Your Own Fan Club

*H*ow would you feel if everywhere you turned, people showered you with encouragement and support? No goal would seem impossible. If you ask children what they would like to be when they grow up, they do not impose any restrictions on themselves. They believe they can do anything because no one has told them that they cannot. But as we grow up, we are exposed to other people's perceptions and beliefs about us, and these begin to shape our view of ourselves.

A case in point is Amy, a first-year university student who wanted to be a writer. She received As in English throughout high school and wrote many short stories on her own. She loved to read novels and looked forward to learning more in university about writing.

After she received a D on her first English paper, she began to question her abilities. She made an appointment with her English professor to ask what was wrong with the paper and whether she could rewrite it to receive a better grade. The professor proceeded to tell her that he did not know how she had gotten through high school with her poor writing skills and that he had seen eighth graders who wrote better papers. She asked what she could do to improve her paper, but all he told her was that she had one week to rewrite it and that she had better reconsider her ambitions to become a writer. Amy was devastated. She finished the course, received a final mark of C, and never took another English course.

Fifteen years later, encouraged by her husband, friends, and colleagues,

Amy took up writing again. She now has two published books and writes for numerous well-known magazines around the world. It was only after she told people about her desire to become a writer that they lent their support and encouragement. Every time she expressed doubt about her ability to write, someone encouraged her to keep on trying.

To reach any goal we need the support and encouragement of those around us. Many of us are embarrassed to tell others that we are trying to change our diet or exercise habits. We do not want anyone to know in case we fail. We worry that failure will affect the way other people think about us. But by keeping our goals secret we are laying the groundwork for failure.

Why do we — either consciously or unconsciously — lay the groundwork for failure before we have even begun? The answer is simple: because we know from the beginning that we are not going to stick with lifestyle changes and we want a way out. Some people prefer not to tell anyone about their goals because they place a high value on privacy. But most of us have someone we can trust and confide in. These people are our safety net. They are there to catch us when we fall, and to remind us that occasional lapses do not add up to failure. If we do not tell other people what we need to succeed, they can never give it to us!

If you keep your goals a secret, no one will be able to provide you with the support you are going to need. The more support you get, the more likely you will be to reach your goals successfully. "No man is an island unto himself" is especially true when you are trying to change habits you have had for years.

Family, friends, and co-workers are your three main sources of support. They can form your fan club and cheer you on to success. These people will help you stay on track and keep you going when you feel you just want to give up. You will be surprised at how many of your supporters will tell you that they are going through similar lifestyle changes in their own lives.

Change can be an unpredictable and lonely process. Telling people what you need and sharing your feelings with them reinforces your relationships and gains you allies. Moreover, if other people know what you are doing and support you during your lifestyle change, you may motivate and inspire them to change their unhealthy habits.

How to Get Your Family Behind You

*Y*our family is the core of your life. The times you spend together are like raindrops on a pond. One raindrop creates a ripple that causes motion in the rest of the pond. One family member's actions or habits cause a ripple affect through the rest of the family. These actions can be subtle (your husband places a bowl of potato chips on the table in front of you when he knows you are trying to change the types of food you eat) or they can be overt (your son asks to be driven somewhere just when you normally take a walk). When you are trying to change your lifestyle, your family needs to be fully aware of what you are trying to accomplish, why your goals are important to you, and what you need from them to ensure your success.

Often when we are trying to make lifestyle changes, we do not include our families in the process. We prepare the same meals we prepared for them in the past while cooking something different for ourselves. This simply does not make sense. Besides the added cost and time to prepare two separate meals, we have difficulty watching our families eat a meal we know is not the best choice. Feelings of isolation from the family only make change more difficult. If we know we should eat healthier meals, why wouldn't we want our families to do the same? Smaller portions and dishes that are low in fat will be good for everyone.

The first step to getting your family members behind you is to explain the lifestyle changes you want to make. Start by telling them what you would like to do and when you are going to start making changes. Explain how these changes may affect your health in the short and long term, and why you feel you need to make them. Then tell your family what you need from them: anything from encouragement and support, to keeping junk food outside the house. They must also understand and respect that the time that you have scheduled to exercise is your non-negotiable personal time. Finally, you should emphasize that you are going to try your best to make these changes permanent. Nevertheless, you are only human and at times you may be sidetracked from your goals. A gentle nudge or kind word — rather than criticism or reproaches — would help to remind you of how important these changes are.

One way to get your family on board with your chosen lifestyle changes is to ask them to actively participate in the process. Involve them in your life by educating them about their own food choices. If you anticipate grumbling from your children about eating healthier meals, ask them each to come up with a healthy recipe they think they might like. Run a contest to see who can find the healthiest and best-tasting meal. The contest could run for a week or two with each family member submitting one or two choices a week and, if they are old enough, preparing them. This is a great way to experiment with new foods and can make for interesting — and sometimes hilarious — meal-times. Choose a prize that is appropriate and motivating according to your children's ages.

You can also involve your family when trying to incorporate exercise into your life. Ask your spouse to accompany you on walks. If he or she cannot come with you every time, ask one of your children. Find out who is interested in coming with you and set up a schedule of walking partners for different days of the week. You and the person you are walking with will not only attain a higher level of fitness, you will gain an opportunity to spend quality time with someone you love. If walking does not interest you, consider swimming at your local aquatic centre, or try bicycling together. Small children can sit in a carrier seat or in a small trailer hitched on to your bike.

Friends or Saboteurs?

Friends can be a source of inspiration or can make your chosen lifestyle changes more difficult. Most people have friends with common interests, activities, or habits. Think about the friends you most often spend time with and ask yourself what activities you do with them. Do you play bridge, play golf, or go shopping? Once you have identified the activities you share with your friends, ask yourself what else is a part of these activities. If you normally play bridge, what food is most often served? Does eating this food help or hinder your efforts to eat properly? Do you feel that you can choose not to eat this food, or do you know that once it is in front of you, you will be powerless to refuse it? The following Activity Chart will help you to map out the activities and friends that are likely to hinder your goal of healthy eating.

This chart will also help you develop personal strategies to limit other people's influence on your behaviour. Under the Friend(s) column write down all the friends you see on a regular basis. Next, write down the activity that you most often do with that friend. Place an "✓" in the Exercise or Non-Exercise column to classify what type of activity you are doing, and write down what foods or beverages accompany this activity. Finally, in the Alternatives section, write down ideas on how to change activities or foods that make it harder to stick with your lifestyle changes.

Sample Activity Chart

Friend(s)	Activity	Exercise	Non-Exercise	Food
Sue/Janet/Angela	Bridge		✓	Cake, chips

Alternatives

1 Bring my own healthy foods to snack on.
2 Ask the group if we can serve healthier foods.
3 Serve healthy food when the game is at my house.

The person who filled out the above form decided to talk with the other players as a group. She was hesitant to speak up because she did not want to force her lifestyle changes on anyone else. However, they agreed that they would all benefit from eating healthier snacks. They did decide, though, that on the last Thursday of every month they would put out some cake and chips along with the healthier choices. Our dieter was fortunate that her friends agreed, but she was prepared to bring her own snacks.

Take a moment to fill out your own Activity Chart on the following page.

Activity Chart

Friend(s)	Activity	Exercise	Non-Exercise	Food

Alternatives

1 ....

2 ....

3 ....

Friend(s)	Activity	Exercise	Non-Exercise	Food

Alternatives

1 ....

2 ....

3 ....

Friend(s)	Activity	Exercise	Non-Exercise	Food

Alternatives

1 ....

2 ....

3 ....

Friend(s)	Activity	Exercise	Non-Exercise	Food

Alternatives

1 ....

2 ....

3 ....

If, after filling out the chart, you notice that none of your activities involve exercise, suggest to your friends that you find an active pastime such as golf, tennis, swimming, walking, or biking that you can do together.

Friends sometimes sabotage your efforts to stick with lifestyle changes by offering well-intentioned advice: Andrea's friends all knew she was trying to change her eating habits and had said that they supported her. At lunch one day, Andrea felt full after eating a healthy low-fat meal. Her friends ordered dessert but she declined. When the desserts arrived, Melissa leaned over and whispered, "Are you sure you don't want any?" as she took an extra fork off the table and handed it to Andrea.

"No, I'm fine, thanks." Andrea put the fork back down on the table.

"Are you sure? I can't eat all this by myself. We could share it."

"I really am quite full." Andrea sat back in her chair.

"You know that you are not supposed to deprive yourself of foods that you like. You're supposed to treat yourself sometimes. If you don't, it's impossible to stick with a diet. Just have a few bites. You'll feel better," Melissa cajoled. Andrea picked up the fork.

"All right, but just a few bites." Andrea ate half the dessert, even though she did not really want it.

Afterwards, Andrea realized why she had given in to Melissa. She had felt pressured to eat the dessert so as not to offend her friend by refusing her apparent generosity. But with or without knowing it, Melissa was sabotaging Andrea's efforts to eat a healthier diet.

When you are confronted by what you assume is a well-intentioned friend, thank them for their advice, then do what you know is right for you. Some friends may resist your efforts to change because they fear that your relationship with them will also change. If you have a friend who also wants to lose weight, but is not ready to make the necessary changes in her life, she may worry about how she will feel when you have lost weight and she has not. As you become healthier, you will inevitably want to try out new activities that may reduce the time you spend with certain friends. A true friend is someone who will support you unconditionally and allow you to follow your heart. The friends who help you go through the process of change will become closer to you and your circle will widen as you meet new people who also embrace a healthy lifestyle.

Gaining Support at Work

Of all the places that you seek support, the workplace can be the most difficult. Office politics may affect how you feel about telling your co-workers what you are trying to achieve. You may shy away from telling them about your lifestyle changes because you fear a setback or failure will reflect badly on your abilities in the workplace. Make sure to choose carefully whom at work you confide in.

If you have a personal assistant, let him or her know that you plan to make some changes in your routine, such as switching to decaffeinated coffee or drinking more water. If your assistant normally orders your lunch, provide a list of the foods you are trying to avoid along with your new choices. Switch the restaurant you order from if it can't provide the healthy options you need.

Among your friends at work, select someone who might agree to take a walk with you during lunch hour. You will be more successful at getting away from your desk if you make a commitment to meet someone. Make your shared commitment specific. "I'll meet you downstairs at noon if you can make it" is too vague. Say instead, "I will meet you inside the front doors on Mondays, Wednesdays, and Fridays at noon. If either of us is delayed or can't make it, let's call each other as soon as we know there is going to be a problem."

Many companies today have on-site fitness facilities. If you know of a group of co-workers who use the facility, ask to go with them the next time. Going with people who are familiar with the facility and its procedures will help you to feel more comfortable. Do not feel that you have to exercise the first time you go; rather, get a feel for the facility and watch what other people are doing.

Some companies also have employee-wellness programs. Companies understand that a healthy employee is more productive and takes fewer sick days. Ask your company's human resources department to tell you what type of programs it offers and to see if these programs can help you achieve your goals.

Special Occasions and Eating Out

$\mathcal{A}$ special occasion can seriously undermine your attempts to eat properly and its after-effects can ruin your plans to exercise. When you see an anniversary, birthday, or special social event on your calendar, you may be tempted to assume that you have no choice but to eat, drink, and be merry. From our childhoods, certain occasions or events are associated with food: a cookie to ease the pain of a scrape, eggnog at Christmas, chocolate at Easter, Halloween treats, and so on. Most people average one special event — birthday, anniversary, holiday, or vacation — every one to two months. If you do not think about how you are going to eat or exercise during and around these events, you will experience constant setbacks to your plans for changing lifestyle habits.

Thanksgiving, Christmas or Hanukkah, New Year's Eve, New Year's Day, Valentine's Day, and Easter or Passover — whatever holidays you celebrate, they all involve getting together with family and friends. Rushing around, preparing meals, and buying the perfect gift inevitably increase your stress level. In evaluating how the holidays will affect your lifestyle changes, ask yourself whether stress may cause you to eat or drink too much at special events. The best way to stay on track is to plan what you will eat and drink before you attend a holiday function:

- Eat a healthy meal before you attend a holiday function so that you won't be hungry when you arrive and you will be less tempted to nibble the night away.
- Never stand by a table filled with hors d'oeuvres. Choose what you want and sit down across the room to ensure that you have to make a conscious choice to have seconds.
- Decide how may drinks you are going to have before you go, and stick to your plan. Choose wine spritzers instead of straight wine, or avoid alcohol completely. You will be more likely to exercise the next day if you keep your alcohol consumption modest.
- If you know you are going to overindulge, be extra diligent with your

food choices and add an extra workout to your schedule during the
week of the holiday.

- Ask yourself if overindulging is worth hindering your progress and
  reversing your gains.

Eating in restaurants can be a challenge for those of us who are trying to
make healthy food choices. The problem often stems not from the type of
food that is on the menu, but from our perception that if we are going to pay
for a meal, we might as well order whatever we want. But what we want at
that moment may undermine our long-term goals.

Even if you choose the right foods on the menu, you can be surprised
when your order arrives fried in butter or covered with a calorie-laden sauce.
When this happens to you, how often do you return your food? Here are
some tips to help you keep to your diet:

- If you have the option of picking the restaurant, choose one that you
  know offers healthy choices.
- Call the restaurant to ask what your options are for a healthy meal.
  Let them know your order in advance and request that it be prepared
  without extra fats or calories. When you arrive, order as usual and your
  meal will come to you as you requested it on the telephone. This is
  an accepted practice and most restaurants will gladly accommodate
  your request.
- If you are unsure about any sauces, toppings, or dressings, ask that they
  be served on the side.
- Always drink plenty of water with your meal. This will help to fill you
  up and reduce your alcohol intake.
- When you are full, signal the waiter to take away your plate so that
  you will not continue to eat just because your companions are.

Even if you feel these suggestions won't work for you, try them at least once.
You will find choosing healthy options easier than you think, and you'll
remain motivated because you control the situations you place yourself in.

These suggestions are by no means complete. If you can think of other strategies that will work for you, by all means use them.

Healthy living is about balance. It is not about never eating what you want or never having a drink. It is about making the right choices most of the time and choosing, rather than feeling pressured. Whenever you face a choice, ask yourself, "Is this what I really want?" Make sure the answer is an unequivocal yes.

Case Study *Isolation by Choice*

Debbie takes the hamburger out of the freezer and puts it in the microwave to defrost. On Thursdays she always makes cheeseburgers and fries for her husband and teenage son. Debbie then gets out her supper, a microwaveable low-fat dinner. She started eating better and exercising at the beginning of September, and in seven weeks she has lost ten pounds. *Only ten more pounds to go*, she thinks as she starts to fry the hamburgers.

When supper is ready, she calls her husband and son to the table. They begin to eat while Debbie transfers her reheated prepackaged meal onto a plate. As she walks over to the table she sighs at how good the burgers and fries smell.

The next week is Halloween and Debbie places the treats in a bowl for the neighbourhood kids. All week long, she has been dipping into the Halloween stash and snacking on the mini chocolate bars. *It's not as if I'm eating regular-sized chocolate bars*, she tells herself. *A few minis won't make any difference.*

Debbie works at a downtown marketing firm. She hasn't told any of her co-workers, including her own assistant, that she has started to exercise and eat healthier foods. Every morning her assistant brings in Debbie's coffee with cream and sugar and an apple danish. Debbie always drinks the coffee (although at home she now drinks it with skim milk) and eats only half of the danish. On Fridays, she goes out to lunch at a local restaurant with a group from work. They always order the same things: egg or tuna salad sandwiches or chicken fingers. Debbie doesn't want to draw attention to herself by questioning the waiter about other dishes on the menu, so she sticks with her regular order, thinking she'll just eat less at dinner.

Thanksgiving is approaching quickly and Debbie notices that the weight is not coming off as fast as it had during the previous weeks. She is beginning to feel discouraged. However, she keeps her feelings to herself because she hasn't told anyone of her plans to lose weight.

Debbie has already missed two workouts because she's preparing to have her brother's and sisters' families over for Thanksgiving Day. They usually eat a traditional turkey dinner with gravy and all the trimmings, and pumpkin and apple pie for dessert. Debbie is looking forward to the holiday: there's no way she is even going to think about healthy eating — after all, it's Thanksgiving!

After Thanksgiving, Debbie has a hard time getting back into her exercise schedule and eating properly. While she hasn't gained any of her weight back, she hasn't lost any more, either. She worries that maybe she can't lose any more weight, but quickly pushes that thought aside and goes for a walk.

Debbie's birthday is December 8, and her husband has arranged to celebrate it at their favourite restaurant with some friends. Debbie orders her favourite meal — steak in béarnaise sauce and Caesar salad — and drinks more than she should. When her plate arrives, she realizes that she really doesn't want to eat her meal. Nevertheless, she finishes it off. She doesn't want to disappoint her husband, who has arranged the whole evening, or put a damper on everyone's fun. She gamely eats a slice of birthday cake and doesn't say no when her friend's husband tops up her wineglass for the third time. When she gets on the scale a few days later, Debbie has gained back four pounds — and the Christmas party season is just beginning.

Debbie's first mistake was keeping her goals to herself. She cooked one meal for her family and another for herself. She found that watching them eat the foods she was denying herself weakened her resolve. Although her husband and son sensed that she was trying to lose weight, they never thought about encouraging her because she did not tell them how important it was to her. They thought she was succeeding with her plan because she never said that she wasn't or that she needed their help. Debbie also failed to tell any of her friends and co-workers what she was trying to accomplish, so she had no one to talk to when she was feeling discouraged. She allowed them to become unwitting saboteurs who urged her to drink more or to eat that fat-laden apple danish. Debbie also used holidays and celebrations as automatic "time outs" from her plan. She overindulged when, with a little planning, she could have enjoyed herself and still have reached her goals.

Ten Key Steps to Success

To increase your chances of reaching your goals, you need the support and encouragement of your friends and family. You have to tell them not only what you are doing, but why you are doing it and what you will need from them in order to succeed. When you have a good network of people supporting you, you will feel more motivated to persevere.

You should also start thinking proactively about the situations that you will be in — such as eating in restaurants and enjoying holidays — and how you can still enjoy your time with family and friends while remaining true to yourself and your goals. Once you begin to plan in advance how you will handle potential problems, you will find that the right decisions soon become automatic.

1 Decide how comfortable you are telling people about your lifestyle changes. If you feel uncomfortable, ask yourself if you feel truly committed to these changes.

2 Always actively involve your family in your changes. Tell them what you are doing, why you are doing it, and how they can help.

3 Fill out the Activity Chart. Evaluate what you do with which friends and decide whether you need to change any activities.

4 Tell your friends what you are doing and suggest ways they can help you. Thank friends who offer advice, but do what is best for you.

5   Advise the people closest to you at work about the specific changes you are trying to make regarding your eating habits or exercise.

6   Do not use holidays as time outs from your commitment to lead a healthier lifestyle.

7   Never go to a cocktail party on an empty stomach, and don't hang out next to the food.

8   Call restaurants in advance and ask about their healthy meal choices. Always ask how a meal is prepared.

9   If you are unsure about a sauce or a dressing in a restaurant, ask that it be served on the side.

10   Understand that the people who truly love you will want to help you reach your goals and make your changes permanent ones.

8

Guilt-free Fitness

$\mathcal{W}$ouldn't it be great if you never felt guilty about avoiding things you know you should do, or about doing things you know you shouldn't do? I am not talking about feelings of guilt about committing a crime or even an act of unkindness, but about how you feel when you know you should be taking better care of yourself. Trying to change your lifestyle should be a powerful and positive journey, not an exercise in guilt. There are several situations that can make you feel guilty:

- Knowing you should change your lifestyle but not doing anything about it.
- Missing a workout.
- Eating too much of all the wrong foods.
- Reverting to unhealthy behaviours.

When we start to feel bad about ourselves, we get stuck, and find it difficult to move forward with our plans for change. To alleviate guilt, we push our thoughts about exercise and eating a healthier diet to the back of our minds, thinking that we'll get to them when we have time. Our feelings of guilt do not go away, they just arise less frequently. But we have already learned that we will never have the time unless we make it.

People who have already implemented changes in their lives feel guilty when they miss a scheduled workout or overeat. Instead of focusing on eliminating these lapses in the future, they revert to their old behaviours. Why don't they just change the negative actions — such as eating cheesecake or skipping a workout — that caused them to feel guilty, and take positive action such as eating properly and exercising? Because it is easier to revert to old behaviours than to deal with feelings of guilt. But, in this scenario, guilt is simply replaced with feelings of failure and a loss of self-confidence.

Everyone is going to miss a workout and not eat the perfect diet on occasion. Guilt is inevitable: you might as well make it work *for* you rather than against you.

You should never feel guilty while trying to change your lifestyle. If you recognize that you are only human and are going to have some good days and some bad days, you can reduce the intensity of the negative feelings you might experience. You often hear that you must have willpower and determination to achieve your goals. Just because you have a bad day and break your commitment to exercise and eat well, do you suddenly have no determination and willpower? Determination and willpower are character traits. If you have an occasional lapse, that does not mean that you have a flaw in your character, or that you can never change your lifestyle. The words "willpower" and "determination" should never be used in association with lifestyle changes. Substitute the word "commitment." If you have not started to change your lifestyle, it is simply because you are not committed to it yet.

If you have had a bad day, it is because you were not committed to your changes *on that particular day*. If you revert to former behaviours, you have decided not to continue to commit to your chosen lifestyle changes at this time. Everyone has the capacity to change, regardless of personality and character traits. Everyone has choices. You can choose to commit to your lifestyle changes, or not to.

One way to transform feelings of guilt into positive, productive feelings is to change the way you think about yourself when you feel guilt. Instead of taking yourself to task, think of the guilt as an alarm system programmed to remind you of your decision to change your habits. Use these twinges of conscience to your advantage. Think about what you would say to a friend in need of encouragement, and use these words on yourself. Be as kind to yourself as you would be to someone else you love who needs your support. The past is history; only the present can shape your future.

Preparing for Setbacks

Life is not perfect. You should not expect yourself to have a perfect transition from old negative behaviours to new positive ones. There are going to be difficult days. It requires conscious effort on a day-to-day basis to stay committed to your new changes. You are going to have days when you are tired, stressed, or simply off your game. On these days you will have an increased chance of missing exercise or eating unhealthily. One bad day does *not* eliminate all the good days that you have had. The question is, what are you going to do now?

You may feel defeated when you have a bad day, but you must judge it for what it is, and then decide where you are going to go from there. First, figure out why you "fell off the wagon." Were you tired? Is a particular situation at home or at work causing you stress? If you can determine why you were less committed to your lifestyle changes on any given day, you can decide how to change the situation so you won't repeat the performance in the future. If you were just tired, think about going to bed a little earlier. If you come up with the answer "I just did not feel like it," ask yourself why. Sometimes you will not be able to pinpoint a reason right away, but you must remember that you still have control over your actions in the future.

The best way to keep yourself on track is to think about how you will cope with demotivation *before* you have an off day.

Let's look at what you will do if you miss a scheduled workout. If you normally exercise on Mondays, Wednesdays, and Fridays, and you miss your workout on Monday, your first reaction might be to wait until Wednesday to resume your exercise. What will happen if something unforeseen happens and you miss your workout on Wednesday too? Most people set their sights on Friday. Can you see where this is going? The longer the interval between workouts, the harder it is to resume them. Missing your workout is like falling off a horse. The sooner you get back on, the better. If you miss a workout on Monday, you should reschedule for Tuesday. If that is not possible, your best bet is to exercise on Wednesday and schedule a workout on Thursday. You will make up the day you missed instead of losing it. Remember, results follow consistency. The sooner you make up the missed workout, the better chance you have of feeling and seeing those results.

Eating the wrong foods on a bad day gives rise to a different reaction. People who have overeaten tend to overly restrict their food intake the following day, thinking they can balance their calorie intake. But this can have a boomerang affect. When you restrict your intake, you will inevitably be tempted to eat too much the day after that because you are hungry — or as a reward for being so "good." The key is to return to how you were eating before you got off-track. If you want to balance your calorie intake, schedule an extra workout that week.

What are you going to do if you have to travel for business or personal reasons? Most hotels have fitness facilities on the premises that guests can use for free, or perhaps a small fee. If you are not used to working out in a fitness facility, allow time in your day for a walk. Check with the hotel about suitable, safe areas if you are unfamiliar with the city.

Vacations are our reward for working hard during the rest of the year. We all look forward to being free of responsibility and indulging ourselves. If you feel that a vacation is going to wreak havoc with your intentions to exercise and eat properly, why not book your holiday at a health spa? Then you can indulge yourself with a massage or a yoga class rather than with food and lazing around. Spas serve healthy gourmet foods and have a variety of activities, so you can get the exercise you need while trying new things.

Your road to healthy living will not always be smooth, but with planning and the right attitude about setbacks, you can confidently move forward in the right direction.

All or Nothing at All

*W*hen people try to change too many aspects of their lives at once, they decrease their chances of succeeding with any one change. Take Sam, for example. Sam wants to start exercising but feels that he must change his eating habits and quit smoking, too. Sam has an all-or-nothing attitude. Maybe he will be successful at consistently exercising and changing his eating habits, but if he has a hard time quitting smoking he is liable to feel guilty. Guilt may prompt him to give up exercise and eating properly. It is important not to try to change too many things at the same time. If Sam's goal is to be healthier, he could start with exercise. After he feels comfortable with exercising regularly, he could begin to change his eating habits. A consistent exercise regimen will help decrease his craving for cigarettes.

People who have had an interruption in their workout schedule or healthy eating habits also use the all-or-nothing attitude. Once they have missed a workout or two they think, "That's it, I can't do this," and revert to their old behaviours. Some people externalize their guilt and blame events, circumstances, or people they think have prevented them from sticking to their lifestyle changes. Others will internalize their guilt and resort to self-blame, believing they are not capable of change. People who externalize place the responsibility for their failures on other people; people who internalize place the blame on themselves. Both patterns reflect an all-or-nothing attitude.

People who have this attitude are sometimes referred to as Type A personalities, or perfectionists. Most often, these people are highly intelligent and motivated to succeed. They work hard at everything they want to accomplish, organize their time effectively, and plan in advance. But perfection always eludes them, because perfection doesn't exist.

To make permanent lifestyle changes, you must be able to distinguish between a *lapse* in behaviour and a *relapse*. A lapse is a temporary deviation from your current healthy behaviours. The key word is "temporary." A relapse is a prolonged period of deviating from your chosen lifestyle changes. If you have missed working out for a week or two, that is a lapse. If you miss working out for two or more weeks and then give up, that is a relapse. The timetables for lapses and relapses are not set in stone, especially if an emotional or stressful event has occurred in your life such as moving, divorce, or illness. The key to distinguishing between the two lies in examining what your intentions are concerning a return to your chosen lifestyle, and following up your intentions with actions.

Everyone who has tried to change his or her lifestyle has had some setbacks and lapses — it is only human. You should not feel guilty about having a lapse. Why should you hold yourself to standards that no one else could reach? See lapses for what they are and continue your efforts to live a healthier lifestyle. Otherwise, you run the risk of allowing guilt to cause you to quit, and you'll end up back where you started, having earned only a feeling of failure for all your hard effort.

Case Study *Say No to Guilt*

David is the oldest of three siblings. At age fifty-five, he has a wife and three teenage children. *Where has the time gone?* he wonders, when he sees in his children the energy he has lost. He has been feeling tired lately and has decided it's time to make some changes in his life. He meant to quit smoking years ago but somehow never got around to it. He knows that smoking will eventually kill him, if his lack of exercise and unhealthy diet don't do him in first. David has decided that on Monday he is going to quit smoking and start eating better. Later in the week, he plans to start exercising.

Monday comes and David quits smoking cold turkey. He has a bowl of fruit salad for breakfast along with a bowl of whole-grain cereal. While David has his coffee he feels his first longing for a cigarette. By the time he gets to work, he feels desperate for a smoke. At lunchtime, he usually pops into the deli downstairs for a corned beef sandwich and a soft drink. Today, he orders a sliced turkey sandwich with no mayonnaise, a bottle of water, and a black coffee to take back to his office. *Not bad*, he thinks, pleased that he's finally making changes.

That night for supper his wife has prepared spaghetti with meat sauce. He eats half his usual portion and refuses the parmesan cheese topping that he loves. After dinner he usually relaxes with a cup of coffee, the news, and a cigarette. Tonight he feels jittery, and his craving to smoke is intense.

David has chosen to start exercising on Wednesday. He has joined his local fitness club and is planning to work out at 5:30 p.m.

David's co-workers have noticed that he is edgy and short-tempered this week. They know that he has a big presentation to put together for the end of the week, but they are still put off by his behaviour, and start to avoid him.

On Thursday, David is sore from working out. He had one more day to get his presentation ready for Friday's meeting. He's feeling hungrier than usual and stressed out. *If I could just have one cigarette I could relax and concentrate*, he tells himself. He knows he'll have to take work home to be ready for tomorrow.

On the way home, David picks up a vegetarian pizza for supper. He also stops at a convenience store and buys a pack of cigarettes — just to get him through the next day. *I'll just have one. That's all I need.* On the way home, David smokes that one cigarette and feels more relaxed.

On his way to work on Friday, David opens his pack of cigarettes. He smoked five last night and has another in the car.

His presentation goes well, but instead of exercising after work he decides to go straight home and flake out. It's been one hell of a week. He hasn't eaten very well that day; he's just been so busy. As David relaxes after supper he has another cigarette but decides it will be his last. His resolve is short-lived, however; he smokes half a pack over the weekend, doesn't watch what he eats, and doesn't make it to the fitness club.

Monday morning David lights up a cigarette with his coffee, feeling strong pangs of guilt over what he labels his lack of willpower. *It's just too hard*, he thinks. *Other people may be able to quit smoking but I can't. What's wrong with me?* He feels his self-confidence plummet.

This is just not the right time to make these changes, he rationalizes. *Work is crazy and I'm so busy with the kids. No wonder I can't stick to my changes. I'll try again in the New Year*, he tells himself and feels a bit better. Nevertheless, in the back of his mind, David worries that he's not capable of making the changes he wants to make. Guilt and self-doubt surface whenever he has a quiet moment.

Five years later, at age sixty, David has a massive heart attack from which he will never fully recover. When asked what advice he would give to others who are trying to change their unhealthy behaviours, David has this to say: "If I had stuck to my changes five years ago, this might not have happened. I tried to make too many changes in my life at once. When I couldn't do one, quit smoking, I convinced myself that I couldn't do any of them. I should have started with exercise and then slowly tackled my diet and smoking problems.

"I did have a choice to continue with my lifestyle changes even after I had a bad week. But I chose instead to turn a lapse into a complete relapse, then persuaded myself that it wasn't my fault, so I could feel better about giving up. My advice is to concentrate on one thing at a time and gradually move on to others. If you have a bad week, so what? That doesn't mean that you can't succeed, because you can. I no longer have many choices of what I can and cannot do. In fact, I have no choices. There is nothing like a massive coronary to give you greater perspective on life and the choices that you make. If you have a choice now, make it wisely."

Ten Key Steps to Success

Our feelings play a powerful role in the decisions we make on a day-to-day basis. Changing our lifestyles should be a time of self-discovery and enlightenment, but too often we allow negative feelings such as guilt, anger, or remorse to overshadow our accomplishments or good intentions.

You already know that you are not perfect; therefore, you are not going to have a perfect transition from your old behaviours to your new healthy lifestyle changes. There are going to be some challenges and some setbacks mixed in with your successes. How you deal with your setbacks, and the feelings you encounter as a result, will either help you continue with your changes or stop you in your tracks. If you can change the way you think about your feelings of guilt, you can move forward and continue with the positive changes you have made in your life.

1   Understand that everyone has setbacks at some point, and you will too.

2   Recognize that having a setback does not mean you are incapable of change.

3   Substitute "commitment" for "determination" and "willpower" in your thoughts.

4   Change feelings of guilt into positive and productive feelings.

5   When you experience feelings of guilt, think of them as an alarm system reminding you of your commitment to lead a healthier lifestyle.

6   Talk to yourself as you would talk to a friend who needs your support and encouragement.

7   When you have a bad day, try to discover what caused you to miss your workout or overeat. Develop a plan, so you will not let a similar situation cause you to repeat this lapse.

8   If you miss a workout, schedule an extra one the next day.

9   If you overeat, return to your healthy eating habits the next day. Do not try to overly restrict your calorie intake to make up for one bad day.

10   Lapses and relapses are not the same thing. Do not mistake one for the other.

Conclusion

*M*ost people's lives, thoughts, and feelings are often in conflict with their goals. They say they want to change, but in reality they are not prepared to change. They have no strategies, tools, or insights into *why* they want to change (beyond the obvious).

If you have read this book and worked your way through the charts, you have by now anticipated your obstacles and barriers and have planned for them. You possess the strategies and tools — along with new insight into what is truly motivating you — to change your lifestyle. You are now prepared to begin a wonderful journey of self-discovery.

A whole new world awaits you. Activities that seemed too difficult in the past will pique your interest. Things you have always wanted to try will seem more doable when you have a healthy body and the increased confidence that comes from overcoming obstacles and reaching your goals.

You now have a choice to make. You can either commit to reaching your goals or you can sit on the sidelines of life and watch others as they change and grow.

I have written this book to help you better prepare yourself for permanent lifestyle changes by gathering your commitment, courage, and confidence and putting them to work for you. These strengths lie within each of us, waiting to be found, brought out, and used.

Believe in your own personal power to change and grow — I do.

An Invitation from the Author

I would like to hear about your experiences with healthy lifestyle changes. Please let me know what barriers and obstacles — or excuses — you have encountered, and what you are doing or have done to overcome them. I welcome your thoughts, feelings, and insights about the struggles and victories in your personal journey, and would like to hear how the ideas and advice in this book have affected you. I look forward to hearing from you.

You can reach me at:

Susan Cantwell and Associates
P.O. Box 591
Station A
Fredericton, NB
E3B 5A6
(506) 459-2665
scprofit@nbnet.nb.ca